AAI-4507

P9-DKF-530

WITHDRAWN

The Substance Abuse Problems

Volume Two
New Issues for the 1980s

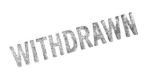
WITHDRAWN

Sidney Cohen holds degrees in Pharmacy and Medicine, and was awarded a Doctor of Sciences Degree from Columbia University in 1976.

Dr. Cohen has researched LSD for the past 20 years and marijuana for the past 5. He has published over 285 articles and 5 books in the areas of psychopharmacology and drug abuse. He is editor of the *Drug Abuse & Alcoholism Newsletter* and is on the editorial boards of *Psychosomatics*, the *International Journal of Addictions, Drug Dependence,* the *American Journal of Drug and Alcohol Abuse,* the *Journal of Psychoactive Drugs, Substance and Alcohol Misuse,* and the *Journal of Substance Abuse Treatment.*

Dr. Cohen served as Director of the Division of Narcotic Addiction and and Drug Abuse, National Institute of Mental Health, from 1968 to 1970. He is now a Clinical Professor of Psychiatry at Neuropsychiatric Institute, UCLA. He consults in substance abuse matters for the National Institute on Drug Abuse, the Food and Drug Administration, the Department of the Army, and the State Department. He has spoken in the United States and abroad on all aspects of the drug abuse problem.

The Sidney Cohen Lectureship, the first in drug abuse medicine, was established in 1984.

The Substance Abuse Problems

Volume Two
New Issues for the 1980s

Sidney Cohen, M.D.

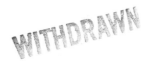

The Haworth Press, New York/London

The Vista Hill Foundation has granted permission to reprint the *Drug Abuse and Alcoholism Newsletters* written by the author.

The *Journal of Substance Abuse Treatment* has given permission to reprint *The Antipodes of the Mind* which appears here as the preface. It was the first annual lecture of the Sidney Cohen Lectureship.

© 1985 by The Haworth Press, Inc. All rights reserved. No part of this work may be reproduced or utilized in any form or by any means, electronic or mechanical, including photocopying, microfilm and recording, or by any information storage and retrieval system, without permission in writing from the publisher.

The Haworth Press, Inc., 28 East 22 Street, New York, New York 10010
EUROSPAN/Haworth, 3 Henrietta Street, London WC2E 8LU England

Earlier versions of most chapters in this work were originally published in the Vista Hill Foundation's *Drug Abuse & Alcoholism Newsletter*, volume 8, no. 6-10 and volumes 9, 10, 11, 12, and 13. Earlier versions of chapters 14, 16, 17, 19, 21, and 24 were published in both *Drug Abuse & Alcoholism Newsletter* and in *The Alcoholism Problems* by Sidney Cohen, New York: The Haworth Press, Inc., 1983.

Library of Congress Cataloging in Publication Data
(Revised for vol. 2)

Cohen, Sidney, 1910-
    The substance abuse problems.

    Vol. 2 entitled: New issues for the 1980s.
    Earlier versions of most of the chapters in these books were published in the Vista Hill Foundation's Drug abuse & alcoholism newsletter.
    Includes bibliographies and index.
    1. Drug abuse. 2. Psychotropic drugs—Psychological aspects. 3. Psychotropic drugs—Physiological effect. 4. Drug abuse—Treatment. I. Vista Hill Foundation. II. Title. [DNLM: 1. Drug abuse]
RC564.C63   362.2   80-21280
ISBN 0-86656-533-7 (set)
ISBN 0-86656-534-5 (pbk. : set)
ISBN 0-917724-18-6 (v. 1)
ISBN 0-917724-22-4 (pbk. : v. 1)
ISBN 0-86656-368-7 (v. 2)
ISBN 0-86656-369-5 (pbk. : v. 2)

Printed in the United States of America

CONTENTS

Foreword

The Substance Abuse Problems, Volume 2: New Issues for the 1980s is a valuable contribution to professional literature. This book will join its predecessor as a definitive reference for the experienced professional. It imparts information and insights to the reader new to the field which will add years of wisdom by careful and understanding reading. The author forces the reader to examine issues in a fresh and clear manner while distilling conclusions from his long experience and the most recent research literature. Beyond the facts, he questions common assumptions and argues persuasively for new approaches.

His expanded discussion of cocaine is useful and justified. Cocaine occupies a special place in this volume. Abuse patterns of cocaine during the last three years have changed the character of drug abuse. Cocaine, the most seductive and reinforcing of all drugs, is now readily available at a modest cost. Casualties are being produced in all segments of society. Myths associated with this menace are dispelled by the author and his concern for its victims is demonstrated in the vigor of his call for a broadly based response to this threat.

A traditional concern in substance abuse is not neglected. Alcohol, society's most abused drug, is discussed fully. Whimsically, Dr. Cohen highlights the denial of problem drinking in his discussion on "becoming an alcoholic."

In the closing section of the book Dr. Cohen shares his insights into the role of drugs in our society. His challenge to the reader is to live a pragmatically based, effective, sober life to the benefit of self and society.

The humane, concerned scientist-philosopher I know and admire is best demonstrated in this book. His intense description of the desire for "the mystical" with a firm rejection of the empty promise of the chemically induced insight is vintage Cohen. His efforts to decipher social and personal factors that enhance chemical responses spares no one. Sobriety, responsibility and the complexity of subjective pleasure are all intertwined to describe the good life. As he finishes the book discussing the future, the fragile nature of the human condition is re-affirmed. The vulnerability of people to immediately rewarding experiences including substance abuse is demonstrated.

Dr. Cohen rejects "pharmacological Calvinism." He forcefully concludes that human organisms cannot sustain "the bedrugged, euphoric state without penalties that exceed the pleasures." He maintains his enthusiastic interest in improving the situation and sustains his curiosity and joy for life. *The Substance Abuse Problems, Volume Two, New Issues for the 1980s* raises the level of understanding and information on this subject into the arena of good literature.

Read, savor and enjoy, Sidney Cohen has produced another benchmark in the field.

Karst J. Besteman
Deputy Director, NIDA
(1973–1980)
Asst. Surgeon General,
PHS (Ret)
Currently Executive
Director, ADPA

Preface:
The Antipodes of the Mind

Using a felicitous metaphor, Huxley describes the mental regions geographically. In *Heaven and Hell* he speaks of the familiar Old World, Europe, as equivalent to the personal consciousness. Beyond the Atlantic sea reside the Virginias and Carolinas of the personal subconscious, and on the other side of the continent, in the Far West with its aboriginal archetypes, the collective unconscious. Across another, vaster ocean, at the antipodes of everyday consciousness, lies the land of visionary experience with its strange marsupial creatures roaming the countryside. This is, indeed, a *terra incognita*, of surreal landscapes to which only a few have made their way, and then only briefly.

It is to these antipodes that occasional strangers have been transported, some spontaneously, and some by psychedelic chemicals. Certain visitors might enter what they construed as a heavenly place, while others were cast onto a hellish terrain to their dismay. Huxley could perceive by the early 1950s that it could go either way.

It is the class of drugs called hallucinogens or psychedelics, and to a lesser extent the euphoro-hallucinogens, that can propel the mind into the grotesque realms of the antipodes. How is this possible? Perhaps it is due to a flooding of the sensory circuitry and a failure of the integrating assemblies. Awareness is, at first, intensified but eventually dissolves. Rational thinking is not possible. The senses fuse, becoming synesthetic. The ultimate mood states are ecstasy or horror, depending on whether meaningfulness or meaninglessness dominates; the final experience is therefore interpreted as either visionary or psychotic.

Other antipodes of ordinary consciousness exist. Convulsions are one. No one seems willing to explore that region willingly, but remember that in certain Eskimo and other cultures, the person who has fits is considered close to God and is a holy person. Coma and stupor are another antipodean domain, and that is a popular place for many.

The use of depressants like alcohol and the others have often been described in terms of survival. "Every culture has its intoxicant," it is declared, implying that a holiday from ordinary consciousness is necessary for humans to endure sober reality, to enjoy, or even to remain viable. A closer scrutiny of this statement indicates that it is not quite true. Admittedly, humans seem to be incomplete creatures that do not cope well with stringent pressures. But the pharmacologically induced distancing of awareness does not seem to improve their ability to do so. Suffering (the old fashioned word for stress) returns undiminished, and eventually drug dependence can become an additional burden.

These generalizations are a prelude to a consideration of those novel qualities of our current upsurge of preoccupation with psychoactive drugs. I also want to indicate what we have learned during the past quarter century.

WHAT'S NEW?

A striking aspect of our present pandemic has been the youthfulness of those in its vanguard. During the turbulent 1960s the psychedelic revolution was led by college students and their relatively young professors. Gradually, the age range of drug users has dropped to the high and junior high school level. The juvenilization of abusive drug-taking has important implications, but the only point to be made at this time is that all previous drug fads occurred in adults. Why this pediatric dominance? Perhaps it is because, for the first time, youth has the affluence and the freedom to indulge.

During neglectful or excessively permissive periods of child rearing, family ties are loosened and often abrogated. Peer influences become the attitude and behavior-shaping factor. This can progress to a point at which youthful leaders of a friendship group are able to instill values well beyond parental abilities to neutralize or counteract what are adverse practices.

The shrinking of parental influence was one part of a general loss of cultural/tribal supports, rituals, and taboos. Other authoritative structures were attenuated: established religions lost many youth to an array of esoteric, charismatic religious leaders. Patriotism was a negative word. However, in very recent years the cycle appears to be moving back toward the conventional.

The culture itself was changing at an accelerated pace, loosening the customary base of stability, and undercutting roots. When the curve of change approaches the exponential, when the teenager's belief system is incomprehensible to the parents, a breakdown of the social norms is inevitable.

The fluidity and changing nature of the drugs involved in our current drug scene are remarkable. Beginning with LSD and its congeners, we moved on to marijuana and the amphetamines, then heroin, the sedatives and the tranquilizers, and phencyclidine. Now cocaine occupies center stage. It is not that we abandon the original drugs. New ones are overlaid and used jointly or sequentially with the old. Meanwhile, our basic potion, alcohol, underlies them all.

Multihabituation, better known by that bastardized word, polydrug abuse, is another new phenomenon. Although speedballs were known in bygone days, most career drug abusers were true to one substance, and were identified after their agent of choice as potheads, hopheads, rumheads, pillheads, and cokeheads. Now garbageheads must be added to the list.

An entirely new event was the development of rapid drug delivery systems. The intravenous route was a century old, but it was traditionally restricted to the heroin user, a social outcast who existed on the fringes of the system. Since the late 1960s, amphetamines, DMT, PCP, barbiturates, and cocaine were being placed into the more accessible veins.

The taboo against using a needle to introduce substances into a vein was strong, and a few people still faint at the sight of an approaching injection. That taboo has been breached by hundreds of thousands of people from every social class in recent years.

The inhaling or smoking of powerful fumes, vapors, and smokes is slightly more rapid than the intravenous route in achieving cerebral penetration. Absorbed over the enormous pulmonaryvascular interface, lung absorption takes only eight seconds to arrive at the brain, half the time required for an intravenous instillation. DMT, the volatile solvents, and cocaine base were some of the psychoactive agents that employed the pulmonary access route.

In addition to being quickly effective, the rapid delivery systems produce a higher peak effect, a highly desired intensity of mood elevation. The decay of activity is also fast; the return to baseline or below occurs within seconds or minutes. Such extreme emotional ups and downs are the cause of intense dependence patterns seen when these methods are used.

One can wonder what the next generation of delivery mechanics will be. The most direct method would be a matter of introducing the psychochemical directly into the ventral tegmentum or nucleus accumbens, the generalized reward areas of the brain. Will technology develop to the point that intracerebral microinjections on the street will be feasible? If so, people will be found who are willing to try them. Beyond that, implanted electrodes in the reward areas loom for those who want pleasure now and on demand.

Another novel element in the present outbreak of hedonic drug usage is the increasing potency of the substances being consumed. Opium, the ancient but still used narcotic of abuse, has been supplanted by heroin, at least 30 times more potent by weight. We know of synthetics that are a thousand times stronger than heroin and are capable of being manufactured illicitly. The alkaloid, cocaine, is more than a hundred times more powerful than the coca leaves from which it comes. This, and the different modes of delivering coca and cocaine make them entirely different drugs insofar as their impact on the brain is concerned.

In the old days, problems were simpler. Stop the inflow of the abused drug and the problem was solved. The post-World War II outbreak of amphetamine abuse in Japan is a classic example. Now we have to cope with designer drugs, items which are analogues of the abused drug, but which are not yet illegal. By the time they are declared illegal, a new series of related drugs are ready for sale. Hundreds of hallucinogens, narcotics, and other drug groups are known, still legal, and readily manufactured for the black marketplace.

I have witnessed, over the past few decades, a deterioration in the motivations for using mind-altering drugs. Originally, the people who tried LSD were generally on a quest for understanding of themselves or their universe. As the drug became a popular item, one heard less about mystical experiences and more about "highs," a demonstration of how expectations can alter drug effects. The LSD story may also exemplify the decay of charismatic movements in general. What starts out as idealism ("If only Khrushchev and Kennedy would turn on together, there would be no more wars"), becomes a psychedelic light show.

The shift from mysticism to hedonism is nothing new, but it does exemplify a fairly normal progression of ideas from the sublime to the ordinary.

Even in the beginning when it was claimed that drugs like LSD were a solution to all our problems like war, hatred, and corruption and would induce instant creativity, love, and the true religion, the LSD theocracy suffered from a surprising lack of a cosmology, a philosophy to live by. Considering how LSD allegedly enhanced the creative process, it is surprising that no broad principles of living emanated from the LSD enthusiasts besides: "Tune in, turn on, and drop out."

While LSD communities were formed, their half-life was less than a year. A few LSD-based religions came forth, the League for Spiritual Discovery being one of the better known. To give you a taste of the tenor of the times, here is Arthur Kleps, head of a branch of the Neo-American Church, another psychedelic religion, in testimony before the Senate Judiciary Subcommittee on Narcotics on May 25, 1966: "We regard (Dr. Timothy Leary) with the same special love and respect as was reserved by the early Christians for Jesus, by the Muslems for Mohammed, or the Buddhists for Gautana."

So, although a charismatic leader was present, the movement failed for the absence of a blueprint for proper living after the established system had been brought down. Its message was too negative, as Houston Smith pointed out in 1966. It suffered from the errors of quietism (drop out), of unselective, fallacious egalitarianism in providing the sacrament, LSD (the worst that can happen is that you will come back no better than you were), of the inability to mesh the psychedelic experience with daily life, and of anarchy, the unwillingness to set standards of conduct and morality.

I have gone into some slight detail about psychedelics because they are an unusual class. For some, the state is so like the spontaneous transcendental experience that an overwhelming feeling of significance accompanies it. It is this ineffable meaningfulness that causes the class to be rediscovered every few decades, and for clusters of people to coalesce around the idea that something of spiritual importance derives from its usage. Such a cluster formed during the 1950s and '60s and included Aldous Huxley, Gerald Heard, Alan Watts, and a few others. A similar cluster developed during the last years of the nineteenth century around mescaline and included Weir Mitchell and Havelock Ellis. Fifty years earlier the Club des Hachichens included figures like Gauthier, Baudelaire, Dumas, and Hugo in Paris. A looser network that used opium as a psychedelic included DeQuincey, Browning, Wordsworth, and Coleridge. There have been other clusters, some long forgotten.

It is predictable that future psychedelic congregations will emerge in time to come, and that unprepared or unstable people will be attracted to them to their detriment. Quick distribution of information and supplies permits anyone attracted to the reported effects to seek out such spectacular effects for themselves. The Upanishads, the Vedas, and the Gita forbid the imparting of higher knowledge to those not yet ready for it. Those who witnessed the fragmenting of some people given psychedelics would agree with these ancient teachings.

A final word about the psychedelic sixties that may sound unbelievable to those who did not witness those halcyon times. It was the oft repeated pronouncement that those under 30 represented a new breed, a mutation in human evolution, and that those over 30 were not to be trusted. These young people would be the generation that would lead us out of our miserable way of life. Only 20 years later this sounds hopelessly quaint, but at the time, it was seriously presented. Perhaps the cycle is closed with the recent newspaper report by one of the psychedelic movers of that day who was quoted as declaring that those under 30 could not be trusted.

WHAT HAVE WE LEARNED FROM THE LATEST DRUG CAPER?

Those of us who watch the scene have learned many things and some of them are worthy of mention.

It seems clear that inexpensive, ample supplies of mind drugs will find people to use them. It is difficult to hopeless to try stopping an outbreak of drug excesses while floating in a sea of that substance. Something can be done to coerce or rehabilitate the involved people, but others will take their place. Is the opposite true? In the absence of a preferred psychoactive agent do people desist from using? Some do, and some go over to less favored chemicals. So supply control is an important but partial answer. Substantial changes in individual and societal attitudes toward incontinent drug use must also take place to achieve a freedom from psychochemicals.

Long ago it was clear that detoxification alone was not a treatment. Few souls are saved by simply removing the psychotoxin from the organism. In fact, it may be that readily available detoxification services tend to perpetuate drug dependency. When drug panics occur, or when the career becomes intolerable, some will clean up the hard way. If easy detoxification is at hand they will use it to reduce their habit periodically and never seriously consider definitive treatment.

As a one time liberal, it seemed undesirable to me to coerce drug dependent persons into entering treatment and to persuade them to remain. I quickly learned that coercion is an intrinsic part of motivation. Drug dependent people come into treatment because their body, the judge, their boss, or their spouse coerced them and implied a disaster if they did not. The ultimate coercion is sometimes needed for compulsive cocaine users. One step back from abstinence, and their worst imagined disaster comes true.

It may seem odd on the face of it that telling people of the dire consequences that will result from the continued use of a drug ordinarily does not affect the drug-using behavior. Many primary and secondary preventive programs are based upon a recital of the dangers and complications of drug use. While potential and actual users have a right to know such information, it is too much to hope that it will deter more than a few. The reason for the lack of impact is the delay in the described punishments and the immediacy of the pleasurable rewards. When smokers are told that over 90 percent of all lung cancers are cigarette-related, it rarely affects their tobacco consumption. The aversive effects are too distant to alter a pleasant activity now.

The factors that defeat prevention are: Easy availability of drugs, friendship group pressures, a lack of externally introduced internal goals and controls that exclude the drug option, and an attenuated authority system that leads to lack of structure during childhood and adolescence.

Successful prevention efforts would require a reversal of these negative elements. It is evident that a social revolution would be needed to deal with these factors meaningfully, a revolution on national, community, and familial levels.

We know almost enough about the wiring of the brain to understand why drugs are capable of entrapping. Two systems appear to be involved. One is the uncovering of opiate, benzodiazepine, and other receptor sites after discontinuance of the drug. This leads to the medley of autonomic and physical effects we call withdrawal, a dysphoric condition which results in drug-seeking behavior. The second is a hyperstimulation of the reward centers of the ventral tegmentum and related structures. This evokes euphoria. After return to the basal mood level, the memory of the "high" induces a desire to return to the euphoric rush. After extended use of the more powerful central stimulants, cocaine for example, dopamine stores are exhausted, and the receptor sites become refractory. At this point cocaine is no longer rewarding, in fact, it may be downright unpleasant. The dysphoria also provokes drug-seeking activity. Transmitter depletion can result in the "coke blues," a painful depression that can linger for weeks after a cocaine "run." Attempts at self-treatment of the depression with cocaine are apt to fail, but this represents another reason for relapse. A final cause for failure to remain abstinent in treatment is the anhedonia, or aphoria, during which the cocaine/amphetamine involved patient cannot even enjoy the ordinary pleasures of life. This, too, is related to elevated reward thresholds from prior incessant cocaine use.

The central nervous system appears to be wired to provide sustained pleasure or brief ecstatic experiences. From the positive and negative reinforcements, pleasure and pain, we learn to approach or avoid, and thereby survive. When hyperstimulation is prolonged by chemical or electrical means, the perception of joy, elation, or ecstasy is lost and cannot be retrieved until the transmitters and the receptors have recuperated.

Thus the hedonic paradox emerges. It is not possible to remain "high" over time; even increased quantities are ineffective in the maintenance of such states. Eventually, continued stimulation is felt as dysphoric or aphoric. In other words, what goes up must come down.

"Escape" is a word often used to explain inordinate drug use. People do, indeed, take substances that distance them from their day-to-day condition. It does not matter whether the life situation is miserable or only perceived so. Sometimes the escape is from some interior noxious feeling. The depressants of the central nervous system provide such relief—but not only the depressants. The stimulants, with their described ability to enhance mood, are capable of removing, for a while, unpleasure.

A good deal has been written about the similarities and the differences between the spontaneous and the chemical transcendental state. But what of chemically and non-chemically induced states of pleasure? While our measures of emotion are much less precise than cognitive measures, it seems evident that similarities and some differences exist. The dissimilarities may be interesting to examine. Chemical pleasures may be more intense, depending on dosage. However, they are often without content, pleasure without an object, as it were. They are, therefore, much more difficult to retrieve from memory since they are not interlocked with some person, place, or thing. Naturally occurring enhanced feeling tones are more sustaining in the period following the experience since they can be recalled and re-enjoyed.

Here is an impressive statistic. Addictive diseases are related to 25% of all deaths in the country. This amounts to half a million people a year dying from alcohol, tobacco, and drug abuse. So we have been talking about no minor matter. Still another equally portentous issue is present. The times demand that we reflect on the question of mind control, whether nationally or self-induced.

We have the technology to synthesize enormously potent opioids without utilizing opium poppies, cocaine-like compounds without coca leaves, and hallucinogens without resorting to peyote cacti or any other plant. Nor would these products be illegal because they are not named in the control legislation.

By the time they were controlled, the psychochemists would have moved on to new and slightly different molecular configurations. The laboratories could close down before the product hits the street. I am describing an enforcement nightmare, a situation that can destroy the uneasy stalemate that may exist at the moment with our drug situation. And yet solutions are possible, or rather, as it always turns out, partial solutions.

Clearly, the potential to alter consciousness will always remain. However, I would like to commend the sober mind to you. With sufficient training, it can achieve even that which is inconceivable. It can transport you to the Virginias and the Carolinas, yes to the shores of the Western sea, and beyond to its own antipodes.

Sidney Cohen, MD

I
THE COCAINE
ISSUES

1. Gift of the Sun God or the Third Scourge of Mankind?

Cocaine is the abused drug whose number of users is increasing more rapidly than any other substance at present. Coca's fascinating history and the freebase story will not be retold here. Instead, the recent research and some ethical issues will be discussed.

RECENT RESEARCH

Although the mucous membrane of the nose is the most favored site for absorbing cocaine, all other mucous membranes, including the entire gastrointestinal tract, are able to transfer it into the blood stream. Blood levels rise slowly and never achieve the high readings found when the material is smoked or injected intravenously. The latter two delivery systems produce an immediate peak and approximate each other in the intensity of the euphoria achieved.

COCAINE—THE ULTIMATE REINFORCER

Animals will work more avidly (by pressing on a bar repetitively to obtain an intravenous "fix") for cocaine than for any other drug. In an unlimited access situation, monkeys will self-administer cocaine by bar pressing for it until they die in status epilepticus. In one study primates bar pressed 12,800 times in order to get a single dose of cocaine. They will work for cocaine in preference to food even though they are starving. They will continue to bar press even though a receptive female is in their cage. They will prefer an electric shock in order to obtain a large dose of cocaine despite the fact that they could have received a lesser dose without a shock.

Such animal "craving" takes place in the absence of personality disorders, situational stresses, or some characterological inadequacy. All monkeys respond in this compulsive manner. If humans had unlimited access to cocaine, they probably would behave in a similar way. The highly rewarding properties of cocaine can make obsessive users of the most mature and well integrated among us.

TOLERANCE AND DEPENDENCE

In the past, tolerance to and physical dependence on cocaine were believed not to occur. This assumption was based on the use of relatively small doses delivered through inefficient or slowly absorbing surfaces (gastrointestinal tract or nasal mucosa) and because of cocaine's brief duration of action. Now that intravenous and smoked routes are employed, very high cocaine concentrations are achieved. Furthermore, the compulsion to keep using is so great that the repeated reinjection or continued smoking of the drug produces prolonged plasma elevations for days. Under such circumstances, enormous amounts can be taken during the binge, and a definite decrease in the euphoria and the autonomic changes occurs, indicating the development of tolerance.

Acute tolerance has been demonstrated in animals; that is, a reduced response from a second dose of cocaine while plasma levels were falling but still elevated from the first dose.

Kindling, which can be thought of as the opposite of tolerance, has also been described. Kindling refers to the appearance of certain symptoms following repetitive, average doses as indication of sensitization. Convulsions in animals have been induced with cocaine under such conditions. In humans kindling has not yet been persuasively demonstrated.

The craving or psychological dependence induced by cocaine is extreme in some people, particularly those who smoke freebase or inject cocaine. Drug-seeking behavior does not occur in all users; snorters are less likely to be obsessive users. The desire to continue to repeat the experience for its euphoric effect or to counteract the postcocaine dysphoria is especially strong when the rapid access routes are used.

Many pharmacologists do not believe that physical dependence (addiction) to cocaine occurs. It is my impression, after witnessing the "crash" or withdrawal from incessant intravenous cocaine or smoked cocaine base exposure, that it does. The abstinence syndrome consists of serious psychic depression, irritability, aches and pains, a restless protracted sleep, tremulousness, nausea, and weakness. Convulsions or deliria have not been reported. It duplicates the stimulant withdrawal syndrome due to high-dose amphetamine discontinuance.

MECHANISM OF ACTION

Cocaine prevents the reuptake of catecholamines, in particular dopamine, back into the effector neurone. Dopamine is also released in large amounts into the synaptic cleft. This produces continued firing of dopaminergeric neurones in the ventral tegmentum and nucleus accumbens in the midbrain. The high firing rates in the reward centers result in the euphoria. Just what the effect of chronic hyperstimulation of the reward centers is, is not known.

OVERDOSE

The LD_{50} for cocaine is calculated to be 1.2 gm intravenously for humans. However, smaller amounts have resulted in fatalities. In such instances a genetic deficiency in plasma pseudocholinesterase might be present. This enzyme metabolizes circulating cocaine. Cardiorespiratory depression or status epilepticus are the usual causes of death.

PSYCHOPHYSICAL TOXICITY

The various possibilities for severe, adverse effects from high dose cocaine use are mentioned below.

Death

Death due to overdose has already been mentioned. Injury or death can result from accidental burns or explosions in connection with cocaine freebase preparation from cocaine hydrochloride. The intravenous mode can produce blood stream, liver, and other infections. The paranoid state has resulted in fatalities because of delusional persecutory beliefs that provoke aggression against the imagined persecutor. Another infrequent cause of death is the breaking of a cocaine-filled balloon that had been swallowed prior to crossing a national boundary. Homicides in connection with the cocaine market are frequently recorded in Miami and other metropolitan areas. Cocaine-related deaths have been increasing in recent years.

Cocaine Psychosis

With consistent dosing, a mild or serious break with reality can develop. The tactile hallucinations, perceptions that something is crawling under the skin, have been called "coke bugs." The misperception may seem so real that severe ulcerations of the skin can be produced by trying to dig out the "parasites." The visual hallucinations sometimes consist of seeing things in miniature, a sort of micropsia. Almost invariably, paranoid thought disorders arise that become very real and threatening. Much less frequently is stereotyped behavior observed. The picture resembles acute paranoid schizophrenia. Dopamine hyperproduction is a current hypothesis of the genesis of schizophrenic reactions. The larger than normal amounts of dopamine at certain synapses with cocaine may evoke the psychosis.

Compulsive Cocaine Use

Two factors drive people toward cocaine-seeking behavior. One is the intense, short-lived euphoria. The second is the neurophysiologic overshoot as the cocaine level begins to fall toward displeasure, dysphoria, or depression. Not only is the postcocaine state an unhappy one, but the magnitude of change within minutes from elation to apathy makes it even less bearable. The freebase smoker and the "mainliner" of cocaine know that another "fix" will cure the dysphoria at least for a few minutes. There are some people who will do anything for cocaine. When this is understood, the compelling need for cocaine is understood. The only thing that seems to stop incessant cocaine use is no more cocaine. When people are so overinvolved in the drug, organized functioning and good judgment are not possible. Impulsivity, irritability, a preoccupation with cocaine, and a flight of ideas make it impossible to think and act consequentially.

ETHICAL ISSUES

Is cocaine a "Gift from the Sun God" as the Incan legend has it, or is it the "Third Scourge of Mankind" as Erlenmeyer wrote during the late 1880s when the first cocaine epidemic was upon us. (The first two scourges, by the way, were opium and alcohol.) Clearly, it is neither at this time. It could become a considerable scourge if we were flooded with low-cost cocaine. Then it is predictable that large numbers of us would be caught up in its interminable use.

Why not use a chemical like cocaine to obtain pleasure-center stimulation? Unfortunately, in a free-access situation perpetual pleasure eventually becomes impossible. The user becomes refractory or so depleted that the question of survival arises. Even if a constant cocainized state could be achieved for a time, it is so disorganized that it is impossible for a person to function. The thinking style invariably becomes paranoid, and this leads to difficulties. Then, when an effort to discontinue the drug is made, the depression can be intolerable.

The only people who do not fall into the cocaine trap are those with limited access to the drug. That, and the poor quality of cocaine today, prevents their slipping into compulsive-intensive use patterns.

Why are we having another upsurge of cocaine overuse now? Evidently, the 35 tons of cocaine that the syndicates send our way each year provide ample supplies for the affluent hedonists. Cocaine fits into the spirit of the times very well. A narcissistic self-indulgence is a way of life for increasing numbers of people. Pleasure now is the guiding principle. Cocaine fits the theme nicely. Pleasure unearned versus pleasure earned: is there a difference? So far as we can tell from the wiring of the brain, pleasure is a reward for appropriate, survival-oriented behavior. Pleasure without purpose is a trick played on the brain, and its long-term consequences are obscure.

Cocaine excess turns out to be a disease of affluence. One hears of thousand-dollar-a-day habits, but these are unusual. However, the average person is spared the disaster of unlimited access. It is the very wealthy person or the high-level dealer who is vulnerable.

The economics of cocaine provide us with another ethical dilemma. Worth about eight times as much as gold, untaxed, and concentrated in a small number of hands, the billions of dollars in this trade becomes a very real human and political problem. It corrupts officials here and abroad. Bribery becomes part of the overhead. Murder becomes a way to deal with undesired personnel. Whole governments have been bought and sold in some countries. What is to be done?

SUMMARY

Little has been learned from the experience of a century ago in Europe and North America when cocaine came forth in a burst of overenthusiasm. It took years for the adverse reactions and the therapeutic disappointments to cause a downward reevaluation of its risk/benefit ratio. Its therapeutic use almost died away completely. It now appears that we are condemned to repeat the cocaine debacle of the past with no more success than the great men of yesteryear—Freud, Halstead, Hammond, and the others—were able to muster.

BIBLIOGRAPHY

- Crowley, A. *Diary of a Drug Fiend*. Sphere Books, London, 1972.
- Ellinwood, E. H. & Kilbey, M. M. *Cocaine and Other Stimulants*. Plenum, New York, 1977.
- Grabowski, J. (ed.) *Cocaine: Pharmacology, Effects and Treatment of Abuse*. Research Monograph Series #50, National Institute on Drug Abuse, U.S. Government Printing Office, Washington, DC 20402, 1984.

- Grinspoon, L. and Bakalar, J.B. *Cocaine*. Basic Books, New York, 1976.
- Mulé, S. J. *Cocaine: Chemical, Biological, Clinical, Social and Treatment Aspects*. CRC Press, Cleveland, 1976.
- Petersen, R.C. and Stillman, R.C. *Cocaine: 1977*. NIDA Research Monograph #13. Superintendent of Documents. U.S. Government Printing Office, Washington, D.C. 20402, 1977. Stock No. 017-024-00592-4.

2. Coca Paste and Freebase: New Fashions in Cocaine Use

Traditionally, coca leaves have been chewed in the South American highlands or taken medicinally as a tea in Peru, Bolivia, and other countries where the bush grows. Coca contains some 14 alkaloids, among which is cocaine, which is present in about 1 percent by weight. The Indians of the Andean highlands describe antifatigue, energizing, and appetite-suppressing effects.

Cocaine is another story. It is being utilized by increasing numbers of people in the large cities of North America and Europe, snorted as a rule but also absorbed from other mucous membranes, or injected intravenously. The parenteral route provides a more intense euphoria but carries with it the risk of added toxicity and the diseases of unsterility. Cocaine is not too well absorbed from the stomach because of its partial hydrolysis by gastric acid.

Cocaine aficionados always have been preoccupied with the routes of administration of their favorite euphoriant. The nasal high is as much as most want, but it does cause sores after a while. The intravenous corridor is a higher high, but it can lead to an obsession with cocaine, to say nothing of a paranoid way of life. During the past few years two new, but related, modes of usage have appeared and are spreading. They are coca (or cocaine) paste and freebase smoking.

COCA PASTE SMOKING

The first report of coca paste smoking came from Peru in 1974. Since then, the practice has spread to Colombia, Bolivia, Equador, Panama, and other countries. Sporadic instances of use are being seen in Los Angeles, San Francisco, and other cities.

Coca paste is the first extraction product made during the manufacture of cocaine from the leaves of the coca bush. The leaves are mashed and alkali,

9

kerosene, and sulfuric acid are added. This procedure produces a white paste or semisolid. It may contain up to 80 percent cocaine sulfate, other alkaloids that are found in coca leaves, benzoic acid, kerosene, sulfuric acid, and other impurities. It is usually sprinkled on tobacco or marijuana and smoked.

A series of 188 cases of coca paste dependency was reported by Jeri et al. from Lima. The patients had complaints referable to their health or had problems of social adjustment. Ninety-six percent were males and three-quarters of them were single. Most were in the 16- to 25-year-old bracket, but younger and older patients also were involved. Coca paste smoking appears to be a middle class phenomenon with the lower, and to a lesser extent, the upper class represented. A third of the treatment group was unemployed. Their hospital stay lasted an average of 12 weeks with the duration ranging from two days to six months.

Those who were interviewed during the intoxicated state described an immediate, extreme euphoria. Talkativeness and overactivity, along with paranoid thoughts, were routinely mentioned. Dilated pupils, a rapid pulse, tremulousness, and psychomotor excitement were observed during the initial examination. Irritability or anxiety, and less frequently aggressiveness, followed the acute phase. In the consistent smokers insomnia and substantial weight losses were noted. Chronic heavy use was associated with hallucinations and delusions. Sexual indifference was reported more often than sexual stimulation, a finding at variance with the North American experience with cocaine.

These hospital patients were uniformly thin, pale, unkempt, and suspicious. The hallucinations were either visual, tactile, olfactory, or auditory, and their content regularly reflected delusional misinterpretations with a persecutory content. During the longer term evaluation some of the patients developed full-blown paranoid psychoses or extreme pathological jealousy. Three patients in the series died, two of cardiac arrhythmias and one patient committed suicide.

The most notable aspect of the clinical picture was the enormous compulsion to continue smoking coca paste until supplies were completely consumed. This urgent need to keep using the paste might begin after the first few cigarettes and was very frequent in consistent users. The obsession with coca paste smoking led to a disregard for physical health, social concerns, and all other activities not directly related to obtaining, using, and recovering from the inhalation of cocaine smoke.

UNDERSTANDING COCA PASTE SMOKING

Why should an epidemic of coca paste smoking arise in South America and threaten to spread to other lands? In recent years the cultivation of coca leaves and the manufacture of cocaine has become a multibillion-dollar industry. The Western world has experienced a sharp rise in nonmedical cocaine consumption. Supplies of the inexpensive paste have become available to the local population during the past few years. The users are not the same people who traditionally have chewed coca leaves, a much more benign practice. Instead, they were either abusers of other drugs like cannabis or prescription items, or they have come upon coca paste as their first drug of abuse.

Smoking high potency cocaine sulfate is approximately equivalent to injecting it intravenously, considering the sharp onset of action and the brief duration of the peak effect. Coca paste is a great bargain compared to cocaine. To obtain a brief ecstatic state easily and inexpensively is a sure method of introducing the practice into a society. The compelling desire to re-enter the state perpetuates its use.

The more alarming features of smoking coca paste are the fairly frequent appearance of psychotic reactions associated with chronic use and the social and psychophysical deterioration that can occur. These undesirable consequences are an intrinsic part of the abrupt and extreme mood shifts from hyperphoria to dysphoria within minutes. The highly pleasurable and very unpleasurable swing is so marked that a return to hyperphoria is devoutly desired. Thus interminable usage is assured. The concentrated use of all central stimulants can produce schizophrenia-like psychoses. The intense preoccupation with the high can only lead to personal and interpersonal neglect. As indicated, the curve of action of smoked cocaine resembles its intravenous use.

In this country it is the intravenous route that leads to paranoid states more often than when equivalent amounts are inhaled. Intravenous cocaine injections also carry with them the strong desire to repeat the event, much more so than the nasal route. The repetitious exposure of the cerebral neurones to high concentrations of cocaine produces alterations of brain metabolism that provoke distortions of thinking and perception in addition to the well-known emotional changes.

FREEBASE

Resembling coca paste smoking in many ways is the smoking of alkaloidal cocaine in this country. Its popularity is sufficient to generate a subindustry: the production of kits designed to convert the cocaine hydrochloride from street cocaine to freebase (or basic) cocaine. Cocaine freebase is much more volatile than the hydrochloride salt. It melts at body temperature and passes into the smoke quite readily. Naturally, these freebase kits are advertised in our very aboveground "underground" press and they are sold in another growth industry, the paraphernalia shops.

Freebase, then, is ordinarily made by the consumer. It is prepared by dissolving the cocaine buy in water, adding a strong alkali, and extracting the basic cocaine with a volatile solvent. These caustic and volatile chemicals have caused a few kitchen and bathroom accidents.

Cocaine as purchased on the street (at a cost of $2,500–$3,000 an ounce) is only 20 to 60 percent pure. The adulterants are usually sugars like mannitol and lactose, or synthetic local anesthetics like procaine, lidocaine, benzocaine, or tetracaine. During the freebase extraction procedure most of the local anesthetics are carried along with the cocaine, but the sugars are not. Therefore what is left after the solvent extraction is less than the original amount that was "basified," and in a few instances, nothing has remained on the evaporating dish. But what is left is potent cocaine base. When smoked it is rapidly absorbed in the lungs and carried to the brain in a few seconds.

Frequent cocaine sniffing can ulcerate or even perforate a nasal septum by its vasoconstricting effect. Whether consistent smoking of cocaine base will do the same to the lungs remains to be seen. A few instances of bronchitis with bloody expectorate have been encountered, but only over the future months or years will we learn whether cocaine lung is a new clinical entity.

Smoking freebase with its two-minute superhigh evokes an enormous desire to keep on "basing." Again the rapid shift from ecstasy to misery impels many users to keep smoking until they or their freebase are exhausted. This is understandable. After all, relief from their desolation is at hand from a single puff.

The results of smoking freebase, either in a special pipe or sprinkled on a cigarette, are identical to smoking coca paste or injecting cocaine hydrochloride intravenously. Mydriasis, tachycardia, and increased blood pressure and respiration rates are the autonomic effects. The "rush" is sudden and intense. Feelings of energy, power, and competence are described. The euphoric high subsides after a few minutes into a restless irritability. The residual "wired up" state is so intolerable that a heroin habit may be started to relieve the tense and overstrung feeling. Sleep is impossible during a freebase binge, but exhaustion eventually supervenes. Enormous weight loss takes place in heavy users due to the anorectic action of cocaine. Manic, paranoid, or depressive psychoses have been seen. Overdose can cause death due to cardiorespiratory arrest.

IMPLICATIONS

The movement, on two continents, from a less risky to a more hazardous form of cocaine use conforms to a general law. It may be stated as: Techniques or drugs that produce more intense and immediate effects tend to displace those that provide slower and more moderate effects. Many examples of this dictum exist. With reference to cocaine, the progression has proceeded over the centuries from chewing coca leaves to sniffing cocaine to intravenous injecting to smoking cocaine. The difference between chewing coca and smoking cocaine is so great that they practically represent entirely different drugs.

Another axiom is apparent: The higher the high, the lower the low. Freebase and coca paste smoking rivals the intravenous route in its instantaneous, powerful high, but the swing from euphoria to dysphoria is so quick that enormous craving is felt by many consumers. The postsmoking low is very far down. Therefore both the positive and the negative reinforcers are extremely strong.

Coca paste is inexpensive (a few dollars a gram) and may become an important item of illicit trafficking in days to come. By contrast, freebase turns out to be the most expensive of all mood changers when price is measured against euphoria time. Affluent hedonists are the only ones who can afford it.

Even the cocaine-snorting contingent looks askance at freebase users. The up-down roller coaster, the compelling need to keep smoking, the devastating impact on mind and body, the paranoia, the unknown question of lung damage, the increased risk of overdosing—all these and other dubious qualities about smoking cocaine base make it too much.

Does substantial cocaine smoking cause physical dependence? The prostration, depression, and achiness are reminiscent of amphetamine-type dependence, but no major withdrawal signs such as delirium or convulsions have been recorded yet. Pharmacologists have taught that tolerance to and withdrawal from cocaine did not occur. This may have been true at low levels of usage, but when an ounce a week of cocaine is smoked, both tolerance and a stimulant withdrawal syndrome will occur. Physical dependence is much less important than the psychological dependence that takes place when quantities of cocaine are used in the manner described.

Post has postulated that the chronic cocaine user progresses through three phases as he continues to use the drug: euphoria, dysphoria, and paranoid psychosis. It will be interesting to watch the cocaine smoking phenomenon to see whether the progression through these stages occurs at an accelerated rate.

BIBLIOGRAPHY

- Grinspoon, L. and Bakalar, J.B. Cocaine: A social history. Psychology Today, March, 1977, p. 37.
- Jeri, F.R. et al. The syndrome of coca paste. J. Psychedelic Drugs, 10: 361-370, 1978.
- Jeri, F.R. et al. Separata de la Revista de la Sanidad del Ministerio del Interior, 39:1-18, 1978.
- Resnick, R.B. et al. Acute systemic effects of cocaine in man. A controlled study by nasal and intravenous routes. Science, 195:696-698, 1976.

- Siegel, R. Long-term effects of recreational cocaine use: A four-year study. Interamerican Seminary about Coca and Cocaine: Medical-sociological aspects. Lima, Peru, 1979, pp. 11-26.
- Post, R.M. Cocaine psychosis. A continuum model. Am. J. Psychiat. 132:225-231, 1975.

3. The Cocaine Problems

What do regular cocaine users want? They all look forward to mood elevation, call it euphoria, elation, or even ecstasy. Most anticipate feelings of increased energy, accelerated thinking, and intensified awareness. Those who use cocaine to enhance their skills, the so-called occupational users, hope that they will achieve increased strength, self-confidence, memory, and a shortened reaction time. Some people look to cocaine for improved sexual functioning, and others desire intensified interpersonal interactions. Such positive effects are possible to achieve, especially at the early phases of cocaine indulgence. The temptation to continue using is therefore great, especially when one must return to the same difficult world from which one started.

With continued, intensified use, especially if one moves on to the rapid cocaine delivery systems, the situation changes, the highs are not quite so high anymore, and the return is no longer back to one's old self but to a dysphoric feeling of being low, tired, and apathetic. Therefore, more cocaine.

The increase in distressing, displeasurable effects can culminate in a series of adverse psychiatric sequellae, some of which are distinctly aversive, but others can lead to life-threatening behavior.

UNTOWARD PSYCHOLOGICAL EFFECTS OF COCAINE

A variety of psychotic options are available to the chronic cocaine user, although the choice probably depends upon the distortions of brain chemistry interacting with the existing personality structure.

1. An accentuation of the desired aspects of cocaine use leads to some serious problems. When arousal becomes hyperarousal and sensitivity becomes hypersensitivity, it is hardly possible to sort out the real from the imagined, the valid from the ideas of reference. Environmental incidents are overinterpreted. Everything, every random movement, becomes intrusive and threatening to one's integrity. The cause of the poorly defined danger is out there,

15

and everyone is suspect. Such disorders of thought are prone to lead to violence, even homicide. These paranoid states are usually accompanied by various sensory misperceptions. The tactile hallucinations (coke bugs) are most often described. The feeling that insects are crawling under the skin may be based upon the itching that sometimes is associated with cocaine use.

Patients might also describe "snow lights," a flickering of rays of bright white light at the periphery of the visual fields. It is more likely that these are stimulant effects upon the optical system rather than visual hallucinations. They appear to have no mental or physical consequences.

2. The attention span can become so fragmented and thinking so accelerated and disorganized that a picture resembling a manicky flight of ideas with a considerable pressure of speech and distractibility becomes obvious to the observer. Restlessness, irritability, and impulsivity also mimic the manic state. The deficits in ability to attend and in decision making can produce a variety of accidents, including single vehicle accidents without an obvious cause.

3. In addition to a schizophreniform and a manic-like psychosis, a confused toxic psychosis might be encountered. This condition includes disorientation, memory defects, and other organic mental symptoms.

4. Stereotyped activities like pacing, bruxism, skin picking, or other repetitive behaviors are probably produced by larger than usual dopamine availability at certain synapses.

5. As the cocaine taking becomes a career, the enhanced sexuality is eventually transformed into a complete disinterest in sex or to priapism with ejaculatory failure.

During the period of withdrawal from consistent cocaine use, a number of unwanted effects occur. The discontinuance of the drug may be caused by exhaustion of the person or an inability to obtain supplies of the drug. The most important problem during the phase is a moderate to severe depression that can assume suicidal proportions. It may be prolonged and require antidepressant pharmacotherapy. One possibility is that it is due to a relative dopamine insufficiency in limbic structures. The depressive feelings may be so distressing that they become a reason for a relapse back to cocaine in a vain effort at self-treatment.

During the postcocaine period patients may find that they may have lost the capability to enjoy ordinarily pleasurable events. The anhedonia will persist until dopamine homeostasis is restored and the reward centers in the brain have regained their sensitivity to noncocaine pleasurable activities. This resetting of the reward threshold may take weeks and patients should be warned of it, otherwise they may go back to cocaine in the belief that nothing is enjoyable and that that is how it will remain.

Polydrug abuse is common in the habitual cocaine user. In an attempt to take the edge off the tense, "wired-up" feeling, a reliance on depressants like heroin, barbiturates, alcohol, or methaqualone is almost inevitable. Furthermore, these drugs are used to relieve the insomnia and to diminish the misery of the cocaine "crash." Therefore, multiple dependencies are frequent.

It is difficult for the nonuser to understand why, if the cocainist has just about ruined his or her family, health, and social relationships, lost a job and savings, he or she will still persist in snorting or otherwise consuming cocaine. Physical addiction plays essentially no role in the inability to desist. It is the intense craving to re-experience the euphoria and to abort the dysphoric aspects of abstaining that drives the person back. Cocaine reinforces cocaine-seeking behavior to an extent not seen with any other psychoactive agent.

UNTOWARD PHYSICAL EFFECTS OF COCAINE

Complications Caused by the Way Cocaine Is Employed

Snorting (or nasal inhalation) is the most popular route of absorption of cocaine. All mucous membranes will absorb the drug and the nasal mucosa is the most readily available. A rhinitis or sinusitis secondary to the reactive hyperemia is annoying. Consistent snorting can lead to erosions, but only rarely are perforations of the cartilagenous nasal septum seen. When left untreated, larger perforations can induce a saddle nose deformity, but most perforations are treated successfully by plastic surgery. The inhalation of cocaine alkaloid vapors (freebasing) can, over time, produce bronchitis. Whether more serious damage will develop in the long-term user is not known. When measured during a cocaine-free interval, freebasers show a significant impairment of pulmonary gas exchange across the pulmonary membrane. The intravenous route of introducing cocaine into the system is more immediate and more efficient, but its drawbacks can be more considerable. All of the diseases of contamination may occur. Hepatitis B, blood stream infections, lung abcesses, and AIDS are as frequent in the cocaine group as with other injected drugs. The effects of IV cocaine can be counted in minutes and those who want to stay high must inject up to 10 times an hour. Three cases of wound botulism have been ascribed to cocaine injections, an unheard of complication with heroin and other drugs.

Complications Caused by an Inborn Inability
to Metabolize Cocaine

An unusual instance of death may arise in a patient with a congenital deficiency of the plasma esterases that metabolize cocaine. When given in doses as low as 20 mg for local anesthesia or taken for its euphoriant action, its toxicity is unexpectedly severe because it is not metabolized.

Complications Associated with Cocaine's
Sympathomimetic Activity

The sympathetic autonomic actions of cocaine are many and, at large doses, powerful. The heart rate is accelerated and, in susceptible people, ectopic beats occur. Ventricular fibrillation is a possible cause of death in overdose cases. Another cause of death when high doses are used is respiratory arrest. Breathing is first accelerated, then becomes shallow and, later, irregular. Overdose is a frequent result of "body packing," the swallowing of condoms containing cocaine before crossing a border. The massive dose is so overwhelming that even when absorbed via the gastrointestinal tract, a not very effective portal of entry, death can occur before the individual reaches a hospital.

Acute hypertension can blow out a cerebral blood vessel causing hemiplegia or death. Although infrequent, it should be considered in the differential diagnosis of cerebrovascular hemorrhage. The vasoconstriction, the increased muscular activity, and, perhaps, a direct action on the temperature-regulating centers of the brain cause hyperthermia that could reach a level that requires prompt, aggressive, cooling measures.

Anorexia with weight loss is the rule in frequent users. A third of the body weight may be lost by noneating or minimal food intake during a "coke run." Protein and vitamin deficiencies of the B complex can be expected. Dehydration may represent a part of the weight loss. Other symptoms sometimes seen or complained of include nausea and vomiting, a cold sweat, pallor, and a fine tremor of the hands.

Major convulsions are infrequent. In animals (perhaps in humans) these can result from kindling, a sort of sensitization of the convulsive threshold to constant, spaced doses of cocaine. Status epilepticus is much less frequent and is a dangerous development, especially if the user is alone and not brought into a hospital for anticonvulsant therapy.

Complications Caused by the Interaction
of Cocaine with Other Drugs and Diseases

A small number of people with a history of coronary insufficiency have been found dead with a white powder in their nostrils. When the powder tests out as cocaine, it can be assumed that the vasoconstriction and tachycardia produced a lethal closure of the coronary vessels. Diabetics who are consistent cocaine users may go out of control, not only because they do not take their medication and do not eat properly, but because cocaine induces epinephrine secretion with subsequent hyperglycemia.

Cocaine interferes with the antihypertensive effect of guanethidine (Ismelin), perhaps because of its sensitizing effect on catecholamines. It is evident that a combination of either epinephrine or norepinephrine with cocaine produces a potentiation of adrenergic effects. Since cocaine has vasoconstrictive properties, there seems to be little need to add epinephrine to a solution of cocaine that will be used for local anesthesia.

SUMMARY

It is odd that cocaine was considered a safe drug without particular adverse effects. In fact, the evidence from the first cocaine epidemic of a century ago can be cited as proof that it is psychologically devastating and physiologically hazardous when used in large amounts or when chronically consumed. The dangers of cocaine abuse are listed to summarize the possible lethal outcomes of the drug.

1. Intravenous use leading to viral, bacterial, and other serious infections.

2. The infrequent person with a constitutional deficiency of plasma pseudocholinesterase may die following average doses of the drug.

3. Overdose can lead to death by ventricular fibrillation or cardiac arrest.

4. "Body packing" is a risky way to make a living. Peristalsis may rupture one or more cocaine-containing condoms.

5. A person with a weakened cerebral blood vessel may expire from a cerebral bleed induced by acute hypertension.

6. Occasionally, a person has developed a fatal hyperpyrexia caused by vasoconstriction with decreased heat radiation, increased heat generation due to overactivity, and a specific hyperthermic effect on the heat regulatory mechanism.

7. If the grand mal convulsions are neglected, death from status epilepticus can result.

8. Patients with angina are at risk when they use cocaine because their coronary blood flow may be compromised.

9. The paranoid, impulsive, hyperactive person is likely to try to destroy imagined persecutors.

10. Accidental death is likely during cocaine intoxication because of poor judgment and impaired decision making.

11. Suicide has occurred, most frequently during a postcocaine depression.

4. The Management of Cocainism

With the latest outbreak of compulsive cocaine use something new has been added to the problems of treating drug dependence. Cocaine turns out to be the most reinforcing (rewarding) drug of all. The positive rewards of cocaine use are quickly followed by the negative reinforcement of returning to the sober state or to something worse, which creates its own demand for more cocaine. A third compelling desire to continue use is the postcocaine depression, a moderate to severe dysphoria that can last for days after a cocaine "run." A final reason for relapsing to cocaine use is the inability to enjoy ordinary pleasures for days or weeks after discontinuing the drug. This inability to feel the gratifications of everyday life is caused by an exhaustion of the reward center and its stimulating biogenic amines. Relapse is, therefore, frequent, and treatment must somehow overcome the compelling reasons for resuming use.

COMPONENTS OF A TREATMENT PLAN

A specific treatment for compulsive cocaine use is not available. Instead, a number of procedures have been found to be helpful. Some of them should be applied and adapted to the specific presenting problems.

Absolute Abstinence

It is necessary to insist upon absolute abstinence from cocaine use. A few therapists have tried to help patients cut down the habit; however, these efforts meet with inevitable failure over time, and they cannot be supported as a therapeutic goal.

21

Abstinence from Other Psychoactive Drugs

Cocaine-dependent individuals are frequently dependent on some depressant drug: alcohol, methaqualone, or other sedatives. Heroin is also used at times when the patient feels so "wired up" on cocaine that relief is sought from the irritability and tension. The depressant drugs also are employed to achieve sleep when the cocaine insomnia becomes intolerable or at the end of a "run." These drugs must be discontinued, and a drugfree existence required during the period of rehabilitation.

Detoxification

Abrupt discontinuance of all cocaine intake is recommended. A gradual decrease does not work, and some patients will disappear from treatment and resume cocaine use during this tapering-off period. One danger of stopping daily cocaine use is the emergence of a serious depression that can assume suicidal proportions. These people require the protection of a residential setting in a unit experienced with cocaine problems. A course of the tricyclic antidepressants may be desirable; however, most postcocaine depressions subside in a few weeks. Substitution of an amphetamine or methylphenidate (Ritalin) is not indicated. Such medication has been recommended because of a presumed attention deficit disorder in some cocaine consumers. It is most unlikely that abusers have sought out cocaine because they have an intrinsic attention deficit disorder. Instead, cocaine produces an attention deficit disorder. Methylphenidate or amphetamine dependence has few advantages over cocaine dependence.

Education

The cocaine user who seeks treatment is well aware of the destructiveness of the drug use. Still, he or she may not be fully aware of the inevitable consequences of a cocaine career. Although intellectual awareness of the dangers of consistent use deters few from persisting, drug users are entitled to know the predictable results presented as honestly as possible. It is a curious paradox that what starts as a search for euphoria inevitably ends as an effort to escape from displeasure, discomfort, and depression. Users of considerable amounts of this euphoriant have a right to know the likely results of their use, but it cannot be assumed this knowledge will change their behavior.

Family Involvement

The family must be brought into the treatment. They provide historical information that confirms or elaborates upon the patient's story. They require careful instruction in dealing with the cocaine-obsessed family member's insatiable need for money to satisfy the cocaine habit. Some families covertly support the cocainist. Lending cocaine consumers money is a counterproductive, futile exercise. Allowing them to steal the silverware, the television, or the pictures on the wall is not helpful; it is as culpable as providing supplies of cocaine for the user. There must be no overt or covert support of cocaine usage. There is no substitute for firmness in this matter. Limits must be set on the availability of salable items, despite bitter accusations of mistrust.

The family is brought into the treatment to provide information, to learn how to deal with the manipulations of the cocainist, and to understand the role of the user in the family. A dissolving family may unite to rescue a cocaine abuser who is disabled and in need. If the user should become abstinent, it may result in the dissolution of the family unit. These issues are matters for discussion and possible resolution. During the recovery period, an intact, stable family can be a valuable asset to the patient.

Pharmacologic Therapy

The need for tricyclic antidepressant therapy has been mentioned. Likewise the futility of substituting amphetamines, methylphenidate, and related drugs has been suggested. Lithium has been recommended to counteract the euphoric effects of cocaine. Its use for this purpose rests on very preliminary data. Tyrosine, a dopamine precursor, has been used, but the results are difficult to evaluate. If a cocaine antidote is desired, small doses of haloperidol, a dopamine antagonist, may be tried, but whether the cocaine user will take the drug poses a question. For a persisting paranoid psychosis, butyrophenones or phenothiazines should be provided.

Group and Individual Psychotherapy

One or more individual psychotherapeutic interviews are helpful in ascertaining what cocaine means to the users and to help them understand how they became overinvolved. The therapeutic plan is blocked out and agreement is made about the responsibilities of the patient and the therapist. A group of people with dysfunctional cocaine and multidrug experiences can help in providing reassurance, support, and day-to-day assistance.

Almost all cocaine users who voluntarily appear for treatment have psychological difficulties in addition to physical, familial, financial, social, and job problems. Some are in trouble with the law. It will take time to reduce the turmoil in the cocaine user's life so that a new drug-free existence can begin. The remembrance of the cocaine highs and selective forgetting of the lows may continue for years.

Contingency Contracting

At times the prospect of achieving cocaine abstinence is so problematic that desperate measures seem to be indicated. Such a mechanism is contingency contracting. In such an arrangement the patients risk realizing their worst fears if they relapse back to cocaine use. They write and sign a statement to an employer or the police, incriminating themselves of their worst offenses. The letter is secured by the therapist, but will be sent if the patient relapses into cocaine use, or if a certified urine test, which can be requested at any time, is positive for cocaine. If the claim is that no urine sample can be provided within a reasonable time, it is considered positive and the letter is sent. Many ethical questions arise. However, Crowley believes such measures are meaningful and are the only way to prevent relapse in incessant cocainists. He found those who refused to sign contracts did poorly in therapy. Of those who did sign contracts, all but one remained in outpatient treatment and were cocaine-free. In Crowley's patients, snorters were as impaired as IV or freebase users.

Hospitalization vs. Outpatient Care

It is difficult for a compulsive intravenous or freebase user, and some incessant snorters, to remain cocaine-free without being physically separated from the drug. Those with ready access to large amounts of cocaine, the wealthy and the middle- or high-level dealers, also need a period of separation from the drug in a therapeutic milieu.

Some people with a primary cocaine dependence require a short detoxification period from cocaine and the depressant drugs they are dependent upon. Some need hospital treatment for exhaustion, severe psychological illnesses, and a variety of infections.

A trial of outpatient treatment can be provided to those who seem motivated and reliable enough to follow the treatment plan. It may be necessary to see the patient daily at the onset of treatment to maintain contact, obtain urine specimens, and provide counseling. They must also be warned about the emptiness they will experience until their reward centers recover from the cocaine hyperstimulation. They must be apprised of the danger that they will feel they have solved their problem after a week of abstinence.

The Transitional Period

For months, perhaps years, the abstinent cocaine user requires close support in coping with cocaine-using friends, especially when he or she must resume a job in the entertainment industry, for example. The patient should have quick access to the therapist or the clinic whenever he or she feels shaky about remaining abstinent. Sometimes, a short period of rehospitalization is indicated. Certainly, booster sessions that reinforce motivation are indicated to avoid relapse.

Cocaine Anonymous groups have formed in a number of cities. Other alternative support groups are Narcotics Anonymous and Alcoholics Anonymous. Some cocaine-abstinent individuals obtain considerable gratification from forming and leading such groups. There seem to be enough social and experiential differences between cocaine and other drug users to suggest that Cocaine Anonymous may fill a need for some, not all, recovering users.

Alternative Activities

Some therapists have found that general physical reconditioning, including jogging or running, is an important part of rehabilitation. Time-absorbing activities that are desirable to the patient tend to fill a void left by the cocaine career that occupied the person's waking hours.

Certain "occupational" users, those who felt they could not perform or think well enough without cocaine, require a clarification of why they became dependent on the drug to meet job crises or extraordinary efforts. While cocaine initially alters and accelerates thinking and provides a feeling of competence and power, it also impairs the finer tuning of judgment and decision making. As its use continues, performance and skills are impaired despite the illusion that they are better than ever. Retraining is needed so the sober mind is used with confidence to achieve goals that exceed the cocainized state. It may be necessary to learn or relearn how to attend, concentrate, and think creatively.

Nutritional, Dental, and Medical Care

Some cocainists are in deplorable physical condition. They may have lost one-third of their body weight due to anorexia. Vitamin deficiencies are frequently present. Insomnia is another frequent problem. Lack of personal hygiene has produced dental problems that need to be remedied. Injuries are frequent with these people, and they may have been neglected. A nutritionist may be needed for re-establishing a proper diet.

DISCUSSION

Like the cocaine epidemic of a century ago and the intravenous amphetamine episode of the early 1970s, our current predicament with cocaine might have subsided now that the tragic consequences of regular use have become obvious in so many friends and acquaintances of users. However, a new factor has arisen recently that threatens to perpetuate and extend this problem. It takes three years from planting to harvesting coca leaves. A few years ago extensive coca bush plantations were established, and the leaves are now ready to harvest. Very recent reports indicate that cocaine prices are coming down, and the quality of the product on the street is improving. This is an ominous development because cost was a major deterrent to heavy cocaine consumption. If the price falls significantly, large numbers of people who previously were excluded from the market will be able to experience the initial highs and the eventual catastrophic lows of cocaine.

5. Cocaine Anonymous

The number of cocaine casualties has increased so rapidly that many users and their families hardly know where to turn for advice and assistance. At least two cocaine hot lines exist with "800" numbers that provide information and referral, if that is indicated. Another development is the emergence of cocaine wards in a few hospitals.

A further attempt to deal with the problem has been the emergence of Cocaine Anonymous (CA), in what may turn out to be a worthwhile variant of Alcoholics Anonymous (AA). It was founded about two years ago in Los Angeles by a long-standing Alcoholics Anonymous member who was doing public information work for a film industry organization. He saw a number of people deeply involved in cocaine who had difficulty finding help from anyone knowledgeable about the special difficulties presented by the obsessive use of cocaine. At present about 30 CA meetings are held in Los Angeles each week, and more than 50 are active around the country in such cities as San Diego, San Francisco, Atlanta, and St. Petersburg. Attendance at a meeting may vary from 5 to 150 people. It is estimated that 12,000 people attend meetings annually, and the number is rising.

AA AND CA

The similarities between AA and CA are great, as might be expected. The Twelve Steps and Twelve Traditions are guides for belief and conduct in both organizations. The only difference in this respect is that the first CA step states: "We admitted we were powerless over cocaine and all other mind-altering chemicals—and that our lives had become unmanageable." Thus CA expects abstinence from all psychoactive drugs including alcohol. This is not an illogical position when we realize that many cocaine users have become caught up in other drugs, such as heroin, alcohol, methaqualone and other sedatives. In addition, after abstinence from cocaine has been achieved, shifting one's dependency to other drugs is also known. Tobacco and caffeine are not interdicted, probably because they are only minimally mind altering.

Coc Anon, a program for families of cocaine users, has been formed. This is analogous to Al Anon for the next of kin of alcoholics.

THE NEWCOMER

The newcomer to CA may vary from someone worried about how dull life has become between cocaine fixes, to an end-stage user, dilapidated, sick, depressed, and very paranoid. He or she is advised to attend 90 CA meetings during the next 90 days to begin the difficult process of self-evaluation, to fill some of the empty time abstaining from cocaine has created, and to learn about cocaine and himself or herself. The only requirement for membership is a desire to stop using cocaine and other drugs.

At the meetings are others who have been through the same chemical grinder. Newcomers can tell their stories if they wish. They usually find a sponsor who can be called when things get rough, and eventually act as sponsors for other newcomers.

For those who stay with the program, the following elements seem important in remaining cocaine-free:

- the unqualified admission of one's loss of control over cocaine use.

- the realization that outside help is needed to deal with the problem.

- the dropping away of rationalizations about cocaine and the false sense of being, somehow, superior to other addicts.

- the awareness that cocaine (and other drug) dependence is a lifelong illness.

- the one-day(sometimes one-hour)-at-a-time concept of AA is retained.

- the need for spiritual renewal.

The Twelve Steps speak of God. Some people have difficulty with this. The concept is a broad one that can vary from the God of some established religion to an awareness of a meaningful Power out there that most atheists are able to accept.

THE CA MEETING

The meetings are usually open to families and friends and last about 90 minutes. A "speaker" meeting consists of one or two users who tell their stories and what they have learned about themselves, about cocaine, and about

CA. A "participation" meeting involves briefer statements from a number of members of the group about specific experiences, thoughts, and feelings. Often a participation meeting will develop along a certain theme. Questions may be asked, and answers are offered. A leader is appointed to conduct each meeting, but permanent leadership or hierarchies are avoided.

What goes on before and after the meeting is almost as important as the meeting itself. At these times socialization and bonding, so important for drug-dependent people, occur. Friendships are begun, warmth and respect are provided, and abstinent behavior is rewarded. The backslider is helped by the group support. Those in distress are given advice including professional referral if that appears indicated. All of these transactions are informal and unstructured.

At periodic intervals—1, 2, 3, 6, 9, and 12 months—the addict (as he or she is called at CA) is presented with a chip to formalize the period of sobriety from drugs. The number of one-year abstainers is growing. As with AA, the people who devote their energies to helping other cocaine users derive considerable benefit from the activity. This is an altruistic activity that is rewarding and helps prevent relapse in the donor.

It is recommended that health care professionals attend at least one CA meeting before they refer patients to them. The purpose is not only to assure themselves that the meetings are being conducted in a helpful manner, but also to learn the variety of cocaine experiences related by the participants. The extreme behaviors manifested by people compelled to use cocaine so deviate from the social norms that the power of the drug becomes comprehensible. One girl was heard to say that she allowed herself to be treated like a piece of meat by those who had the cocaine. Another told how he snorted white specks on the carpeting when he ran out of the drug. This tells us, more than any scientific article, of the overriding pharmacologic imperatives of cocaine.

Certain guidelines are offered to the user attempting to stay clean.

● Do not associate with cocaine users. Leave a place when you find that cocaine is present.

● Switching to other drugs, or trying to cut down on cocaine is futile. The message is: "stop using cocaine and other drugs."

● Make amends with the people you hurt while you were a cocaine junkie. In that way the shame and guilt will be reduced.

● Examine yourself, identify the flaws in your character, cultivate spiritual awareness. These activities will help prevent slipping back into the old ways.

● Look around you in CA. Are these people happier and more content than your cocaine-using friends were?

- Recovering addicts can help the addict who wants to recover.

- Addiction is a progressive illness that cannot be cured, but it can be arrested through total abstinence for a lifetime.

POTENTIAL PROBLEMS CONFRONTING CA

Overall, CA is a desirable support system for cocaine users. A number of them will stay abstinent by attending CA, others will need additional assistance. There is a risk that, like AA did for years, CA will see itself as the exclusive way to manage cocainism. It may ignore the psychophysiologic aftereffects of cocaine use or not identify pre-existing mental disorders in some of its attendees. It would be unfortunate if CA came to believe that they could deal with the entire cocaine abuse problem in everybody. This possibility seems unlikely since many of the meetings take place in hospitals, and many members have come to CA through hospital referrals. But people with serious depressions or paranoid psychoses need more than CA can provide. It would be unfortunate if psychotherapeutic drugs were lumped with drugs of abuse, and CA rejected their importance for certain cocaine-dependent people. A few postcocaine depressions are so severe and life-threatening that the antidepressant drugs and hospitalization must not be denied such individuals. The paranoid state may last for weeks after cocaine intake has been stopped. Sometimes, it can be worsened by a group's attempts to minimize it. It requires the attention of someone who understands the nature of paranoid thinking and can decide whether antipsychotic medication could be helpful. The paranoid person needs protection from self-injury or other injury caused by misinterpretation of his or her environment. Problems such as these should be considered by the CA membership.

The possibility that control and power over individuals will take place in CA seems remote. The rotating directors, the anonymity, and the distancing from all political and social causes practically eliminate the usurpation of personal rights.

Where large numbers of recently using cocainists are congregated, the possibility that small-scale dealers will attend the meetings and be available for business afterward exists. This has happened in methadone maintenance clinics. It has not yet been a problem in CA, but it bears watching.

SUMMARY

Although some of the terms and concepts used by CA are not quite consistent with scientific thinking, it is believed that such self-help groups can assist in the recovery process both during and after medical intervention. Some people will benefit from exposure to CA alone. Many will attend a meeting or two and drop out, but some will return. Others will need other therapeutic structures. And a few will never make it back from cocaine dependence.

If additional information about CA is desired, it can be obtained from:

CA Central Office
712 Wilshire Boulevard
Suite 149
Santa Monica, CA 90401
Telephone: (213) 553-8306

II
THE MARIJUANA ISSUES

6. Marijuana Use Detection: The State of the Art

The acute, intoxicated state induced by marijuana and its chronic, high-dose use results in a number of personal and public health consequences. Hazardous driving practices while under the influence, a variety of mental alterations, and other effects on certain organ systems have been reported under clinical and research conditions. A number of laboratory detection techniques have been developed to provide information about recent marijuana use. Some of them are so complicated and time consuming that they are of value only for the researcher who desires great sensitivity and specificity. These will not be discussed here. Instead, those tests that have clinical, forensic, or enforcement applications will be considered.

When it is recognized that less than 1 percent of the THC (tetrahydrocannabinol) that is present in the plant material will be excreted by the body, the magnitude of the technological problem becomes evident. Furthermore, two-thirds of the THC is eliminated in the feces and only one-third in the urine. The urine is preferred for testing, but the quantity measured is reported in nanograms (a ng is a billionth of a gram) per milliliter (a ml is a thousandth of a liter). Certain test procedures can measure less than one ng/ml, but for other than research purposes amounts from 20 to over 100 ng/ml are relevant.

During the past few years commercial, state, and federal laboratories have had abundant experience in examining a variety of body fluids for cannabinoid metabolites, usually THC acids and neutral THC compounds. Industry, drug treatment programs, the armed forces, parole and probation units, and coroners have used the available detection methods and found them to be quite reliable.

The two main tests are an enzyme multiple immunoassay (EMIT, Syva Corp.) and a radioimmunoassay (RIA, Roche Diagnostics); the latter has been made more sensitive by recent improvements. These are screening tests and confirmatory testing of positive urines with gas liquid chromatography, a highly specific test, is often performed. The EMIT d.a.u. (drugs of abuse in urine) can detect 20 ng/ml, and the EMIT st (single test) is capable of finding 100 ng/ml at the 95 percent level of confidence. About 60 to 95 percent of all positives on the screening tests turn out to be positive on gas chromatography confirmatory testing.

WHAT FACTORS INFLUENCE THC LEVELS IN URINE?

The first voided specimen in the morning is preferred because the urine is most concentrated in that sample. Gas liquid chromatography or gas chromatography-mass spectometry, highly specific tests, are often performed. A high fluid intake and an increased frequency of urination will produce lower levels of THC metabolites. The elimination of THC does not follow a straight line, particularly in the chronic user. For a few days a urine may have undetectable amounts of the drug; later, a positive may appear without further cannabis use. This is probably due to mobilization of the THC from fat stores.

HOW RELIABLE IS THE URINE CANNABINOID TEST?

Although individual variations exist, the screening test is reliable, and especially so when a confirmatory test is used for the positive urines. Factors that produce variation include body weight, kidney function, urinary acidity, stress, diet, menstrual cycle variations, and level of physical activity.

HOW LONG WILL A URINE TEST REMAIN POSITIVE
AFTER SMOKING A SINGLE CIGARETTE?

When the 100 ng/ml cutoff is used, positives might be expected from 1 hour to 72 hours after smoking. The highest urinary concentration is seen at 5 hours. Of course, much depends upon the potency of the marijuana, the amount in the cigarette smoked, the efficiency of the smoking process, and the person's metabolic rate.

A heavy, consistent user who had remained abstinent for a week smoked one high potency cigarette. His urines were positive for six days. The prolonged positive finding was apparently due in part to longstanding accumulations of THC metabolites in his body fat.

HOW LONG WILL A DAILY SMOKER CONTINUE
TO HAVE POSITIVE URINE LEVELS
AFTER STOPPING?

In one study the urines remained positive for nine days at the 100 ng/ml level and for 15 days at the 20 ng/ml level. After 20 days it was still possible to detect very small amounts of urinary cannabinoids by a procedure like gas chromatography-mass spectrometry.

WHAT DOES A POSITIVE URINE MEAN?

Since THC metabolites do not appear in urine for an hour after smoking and they persist for days, a positive has no relationship to intoxication, which may appear within minutes and be over in an hour or so. It may mean that the person has used marijuana within the past few hours or days. Alternately, he may have been a heavy, chronic smoker who had stopped a week or two ago.

WHAT IS THE SIGNIFICANCE OF A POSITIVE BLOOD TEST?

THC metabolites remain in the blood in commercially detectable amounts for up to 20 minutes. Therefore, they may have disappeared from the blood before the intoxication had terminated. Blood plasma levels are not too helpful in accident investigations because of the rapid disappearance of the THC metabolites from the blood stream.

ARE ANY LABORATORY METHODS AVAILABLE THAT CORRELATE WITH THE "STONED" STATE?

A saliva test (Receptor Research Institute) has already been approved by the FDA. It is positive from immediately after smoking until about five hours later. A breath test is under development. It remains positive during and for three or four hours after smoking. It should not be expected that the breath test will be as simple or have as direct a relationship to intoxication as the breath test for alcohol. Both the saliva and the breath tests depend upon the local deposition of marijuana smoke on the mucous membranes during smoking. THC is so insoluble that it precipitates out on the moist lining of the oropharynx as it passes by. Both tests might remain positive even after a meal is eaten.

CAN PASSIVE INHALATION PRODUCE DETECTABLE LEVELS OF THC METABOLITES?

Being in the presence of marijuana smokers, even in a closed, small room or in an unventilated auto is most unlikely to produce a positive urine in a nonsmoker. Only one of 48 urines collected from non-smokers from three to

12 hours during and after close contact with four smokers was positive, and it contained less than 40 ng/ml. Repeating the experiment for three consecutive days never produced a positive at the 100 ng/ml level. None of the passive inhalers reported feeling "high."

IN MARIJUANA-SMOKING MOTHERS DOES THC CROSS OVER INTO THE NURSING INFANT?

Two nursing mothers had positive urines at the 100 ng/ml level while smoking marijuana of unknown concentration daily. Their infants had negative urines. Fecal samples from one infant had significant cannabinoid quantities. It may be that in the newborn, the gastrointestinal elimination route is favored. Animal studies have demonstrated the passage of THC metabolites across the placenta and in the maternal milk.

IS THE 100 NG/ML LEVEL SATISFACTORY?

The 100 ng/ml cutoff point is considered too high by some authorities and they recommend that it should be reduced to 20 or 50 ng/ml. However, it has the advantage of practically eliminating the possibility of a false positive. It is true that some people who have smoked recently will not be detected, so that false negatives are likely. The 100 ng/ml level also rules out the possibility of the passive smoker being found positive. For legal purposes it seems preferable to set the cutoff level a little higher than a little lower.

WHAT IF THE MARIJUANA IS SWALLOWED?

Eating marijuana is a less efficient way to achieve a marijuana effect. About three times as much must be swallowed in order to obtain an effect equivalent to smoking. Absorption is delayed for an hour or more, and it is incomplete. After swallowing, marijuana will begin to appear in the urine beginning 60 minutes later.

WHO SHOWS HIGHER URINE LEVELS AFTER SMOKING THE SAME AMOUNT: THE DAILY USER OR THE INFREQUENT USER?

The daily user, due partly to more efficient metabolism of THC and due partly to fat store saturation, will show higher urine levels.

DO ANY OTHER DRUGS GIVE A FALSE POSITIVE TEST FOR THC METABOLITES?

None are known.

ARE ANY DRUGS KNOWN THAT WILL MAKE A POSITIVE FOR THC METABOLITES NEGATIVE?

None are known.

SUMMARY

The urine test, the procedure currently in greatest use, is rapidly done, relatively inexpensive, and reasonably accurate. If a confirmatory test is added, its accuracy approaches that of most other biomedical tests in general use. It is an indicator of recent use (more than one or two hours after smoking). It does not correlate with the degree of intoxication at all. After discontinuing a daily habit, the test may remain positive for days or weeks.

The technology is available if a zero level of marijuana in the blood or urine is desired. This might occur in high security risk instances, or when extreme precision is required for performing certain tasks.

BIBLIOGRAPHY

- Clinical Summary Addendum. EMIT d.a.u. and Emit st Urine Cannabinoid Assays. Syva Co., Palo Alto, CA 94304, 1982.
- Marijuana and the EMIT cannabinoid assay. Syva Co., Palo Alto, CA 94304, 1981.
- N.I.D.A. Research Monograph Series No. 7. Cannabinoid Assays in humans. Ed.: R. Willette. N.I.D.A. Rockville, MD 1976.
- N.I.D.A. Research Monograph Series No. 42. The Analysis of Cannabinoids in Biological Tissues. Ed.: R.L. Hawks, N.I.D.A., Rockville, MD, 1982.

7. Marijuana:
Pulmonary Issues

From a health standpoint it is unfortunate that smoking marijuana is the common mode of introducing it into the body. The leaves and flowering tops of cannabis sativa contain some 400 organic compounds that have already been identified. When these are combusted, a series of chemical rearrangements occur, and they are delivered to the lungs as smoke. The smoke contains a large number of gases and suspended particles.

Tobacco smoke is comparable to cannabis smoke with two exceptions: nicotine is present in tobacco, and the various cannabinoids are contained in cannabis. Otherwise, an analysis of two cigarettes, one marijuana and the other tobacco, produces roughly similar compounds. Tables 7–1 and 7–2 from Hoffmann et al.[1] provide a list of the major components.

CARCINOGENESIS

Cilia toxic agents, carcinogens, and cocarcinogens are among those gases listed in the tables. Of particular interest are the naphthalenes, benz(a)anthracene, benzo(a)pyrene, and the nitrosamines. Approximately equal amounts of the nitrosamines are present in the gas phase, but the naphthalenes, benz(a)anthracene, and benzo(a)pyrene are present in marijuana smoke in amounts 50 to 100 percent greater than in tobacco smoke. These are all carcinogens, with benzo(a)pyrene being a strong cancer initiator.

It should be noted that the tobacco cigarettes analyzed were formulated from an eight-year-old blend and represent a high-tar cigarette. Since then, tobacco manufacturers have selectively bred strains of tobacco plants with lower tar contents. When dried, plant material is pyrolized, a series of poly-aromatic hydrocarbons (PAHs), like benzo(a)pyrene and the anthracenes are formed. Incomplete combustion encourages formation of PAHs, and the poorer combustibility of cannabis as compared to tobacco probably explains its higher PAH values.

Table 7–1
Gas Phase Analysis

Compounds	Marijuana Cigarette	Tobacco Cigarette
Carbon Monoxide (Vol.%)	3.99	4.58
(mg)	17.6	20.2
Carbon Dioxide (Vol.%)	8.27	9.38
(mg)	57.3	65.0
Ammonia (μg)	228	198
HCN (μg)	532	498
Isoprene (μg)	83	310
Acetaldehyde (μg)	1,200	980
Acetone (μg)	443	578
Acrolein (μg)	92	85
Acetonitrile (μg)	132	123
Benzene (μg)	76	67
Toluene (μg)	112	108
Dimethylnitrosamine (ng)	75	84
Methylethylnitrosamine (ng)	27	30

From Hoffmann et al., 1975

Table 7–2
Particulate Matter Analysis

Particulate Matter	Marijuana Cigarette	Tobacco Cigarette
Phenol (μg)	76.7	138.5
o-Cresol (μg)	17.9	24
m-,p-cresol (μg)	54.4	65
2,4 and 2,5 dimethylphenol (μg)	6.8	14.4
Cannabidiol (μg)	190	–
Δ^9 THC (μg)	820	–
Cannibinol (μg)	400	–
Nicotine (μg)	–	2,850
Naphthalene (μg)	3,000	1,200
1-methyl Naphthalene (ng)	6,100	3,600
2-methyl Naphthalene (ng)	3,600	1,400
Benz(a)anthracene (ng)	75	43
Benzo(a)pyrene (ng)	31	22.1

From Hoffmann et al., 1975

Although Hoffmann and his group spoke of the qualitative similarity of tobacco and cannabis, Novotny et al.[2] did a more detailed analysis of the PAHs and reported that some higher molecular weight PAHs were identified in marijuana smoke that were not present in tobacco smoke. The carcinogenic potential of these newly found PAHs has not yet been determined.

It is well known that cancer-causing chemicals must be activated before cancers can be produced. The enzyme that activates PAHs is aryl hydrocarbon hydroxylase (AHH). It has been found that AHH is induced by the PAHs absorbed in tobacco and marijuana smokes. This means that not only are carcinogens present in both smoked substances, but that PAHs induce the enzymes that will activate them.

It is obvious that a larger quantity of tobacco smoke enters the mouth and upper airways, since most users puff on a pack or more of cigarettes a day. This should result in a higher risk from cigarette smoking. However, two factors tend to equalize the risks involved. First, typical cigarette smokers either do not inhale the smoke into the bronchial passages, or if they do, it is for short periods of time. In contrast, the usual method of smoking marijuana is to inhale the material as deeply as possible, keep it in the lower airways, and exhale only when another breath must be drawn. At times the inhalation is so complete, that no smoke is detectable in the exhaled air. The second factor is the increasing quantity of marijuana cigarettes smoked by individuals in recent years. In surveys conducted in 1979, one in six senior high school students were daily marijuana users. In our study at UCLA the average daily consumption in a free choice situation was 5.4 marijuana cigarettes a day. It could be hoped that with the increased potency of marijuana sold today that less would be smoked because the present material is 3 to 10 times stronger than the usual Mexican marijuana that contained 1 percent THC. This does not seem to be taking place; users are "stoned" for longer periods during the day.

BIOASSAYS FOR CARCINOGENICITY

One assay to determine the carcinogenic potential of tobacco tars is application of tobacco condensate to mouse skin. Marijuana smoke condensate was applied to mice for five days by Cottrell et al.[3] They observed metaplasia of the sebaceous glands, an effect that correlates well with its carcinogenicity. Hoffman's group[1] painted marijuana and tobacco smoke condensate on mice for 74 weeks. They saw tumors in both groups of animals, with a larger number in the tobacco group.

Using explants of human lung tissue exposed to either tobacco or cannabis smoke, the Leuchtenbergers[4] found cellular abnormalities, alterations in DNA content and in chromosome number. They then employed hamster lung explants because of their longer survival time and noted malignant transformation after three to six months' exposure to both tobacco and marijuana smoke. When the malignant cells were injected into mice, fibrosarcomas developed. Marijuana smoke produced the changes more readily than the tobacco smoke. In this experiment the smoke from both plants acted as a tumor accelerator, nor an initiator, since the control group also developed malignant tumors over a 12- to 24-month period.

HUMAN EXPERIENCE WITH CANNABIS AND CANCER

What can be said of the actual production of cancers by cannabis in people? Studies of small numbers of chronic Jamaican, Costa Rican, and Greek cannabis users have not revealed instances of lung cancer. However, although bronchogenic cancer occurs almost exclusively among smokers, the incidence is not great enough to prove a cause-effect relationship for cannabis in studies utilizing small populations and not including information on those too ill to participate in the survey.

Of interest is the experience of a group of American soldiers stationed in Europe.[5] They had access to hashish at relatively low cost, and some smoked considerable amounts. A number required hospitalization for respiratory infections and volunteered for bronchial biopsies. Of the 30 who underwent biopsies 23 were also cigarette users. All 23 had one or more pathological alterations consisting of either atypical cells, basal cell hyperplasia, or squamous cell metaplasia. Two of seven hashish smokers who did not use tobacco and one of three tobacco but not hashish users showed such pathological changes. Of three nonsmokers who were biopsied none demonstrated any abnormalities. The histopathologic lesions found in this group are identical to those associated with the later development of carcinoma of the lung when it occurs.

INFLAMMATORY CHANGES

In doses equivalent to what heavy, chronic smokers would inhale, Fleishman et al.[6] reported that inflammatory granuloma appeared in rats exposed to marijuana smoke for 360 days. The article on American soldiers in Europe mentioned earlier described bronchitis, asthma, and rhinopharyngitis as the reasons for hospitalization. Bronchitis is a common clinical observation in the older literature on cannabis. Mild narrowing of the airways has been noted in a number of studies. A decrease in alveolar macrophage activity against standard bacterial challenges was seen by McCarthy.[7] The pulmonary macrophage is an important part of the defenses against lung infections. The mag-

nitude of these changes is approximately that of equivalent amounts of tobacco smoke. An exception to this is the investigation of Tashkin and his
colleagues.[8] They compared 75 chronic marijuana smokers and controls
matched with respect to anthropometric characteristics and tobacco smoking
habits. Chronic use was defined as at least five years' experience, using at
least four times weekly during the six months before the study. Nontobacco
marijuana users were then matched with nonmarijuana tobacco smokers who
consumed at least 16 cigarettes a day. Specific airway conductance was significantly lower and airway resistance was significantly higher in the marijuana group. The researchers believe that these findings are suggestive that
the chronic use of marijuana in young individuals produces narrowing of the
larger airways that is not detectable in those smoking tobacco.

The narrowing of the airway found with chronic use of cannabis is opposite
to its acute effects. Marijuana or THC, whether consumed or inhaled in single
doses, will dilate the bronchial tree. When smoked consistently, the irritant
and inflammatory changes become dominant and bronchoconstriction supervenes.

JOINT CANNABIS-TOBACCO USE

Smoking both cannabis and tobacco is a very common practice. It is not
known whether the combined use is additive or supraadditive insofar as carcinogenicity of inflammatory reactions is concerned. Nevertheless, there is
good reason to assume that the burden of smoking both drugs is likely to be
greater than either alone. The preliminary finding that PAHs are more readily
formed with marijuana, if confirmed, would make conjoint tobacco-cannabis
use more hazardous than either dose.

It seems obvious that the inflammatory reactions and macrophage activity
inhibition would be at least additive when both are smoked. Therefore, it is in
the subgroup of heavy tobacco and cannabis users that the first evidence of increased pathological changes will take place. Since few people will be dis-
suaded from their marijuana and tobacco habits by a recital of the potential or
actual dangers, it appears evident that another experiment in nature is now under way.

The use of cannabis is greatest among the 12- to 25-year-olds with even
earlier ages becoming increasingly involved. To start smoking either or both
substances during youth will provide a prolonged period of exposure to hazardous materials in the smoke. Therefore, if frequent exposure to marijuana
smoke is a significant carcinogen and inflammatory agent, then we may see
lung malignancies and obstructive pulmonary disease at early ages in the coming years.

SUMMARY

Back in 1912, Adler wrote a monograph on primary malignancies of the lung. He opened his article with the question: "Is a monograph on primary carcinomas of the lung needed?" At that time bronchogenic carcinomas were great rarities. Thirty years later the incidence had increased markedly, and the relationship between lung cancer and cigarettes had been perceived. We are confronted with another popular smoking problem—that of marijuana. When tobacco was introduced into this culture, we had no way of knowing about its serious long-term effects. Now we have the capability to predict that marijuana will be another carcinogen, additive to tobacco carcinogenicity. Certainly, no environmentalists would knowingly expose themselves to these toxic smokes. These pollutants, inhaled into the lungs, are hazardous over time when used alone, and perhaps doubly so when used together.

REFERENCES

1. Hoffmann, D. et al. On the carcinogenicity of marijuana smoke. Recent Advances in Phytochemistry. 9:63-81, 1975.
2. Novotny, M. et al. Possible basis for the higher mutagenicity of marijuana smoke as compared to tobacco smoke. Experientia 32:280-282, 1975.
3. Cottrell, J.C. et al. Toxic effects of marijuana tar on mouse skin. Arch. Envior. Health. 26:277-278, 1973.
4. Leuchtenberger, C. and Leuchtenberger, L. Cytological and cytochemical studies of the effects of fresh marijuana smoke on growth and DNA metabolism of animal and human lung cultures. In: *Pharmacology of Marijuana*. Eds.: M.C. Braude & S. Szara, Raven. N.Y., 1976.
5. Tennant, F.S. Histopathologic and clinical abnormalities of the respiratory system in chronic hashish smokers. Substance and Alcohol Misuse. 1:93-100, 1980.
6. Fleishman, R.W., Baker, J.R. and Rosenkranz, H. Pulmonary pathologic changes in rats exposed to marijuana smoke for one year. Toxicol. & Applied Pharmacol. 47:557-566, 1979.
7. McCarthy, C.R. et al. Effect of marijuana on the in vitro function of pulmonary macrophages. In: *Pharmacology of Marijuana*. Eds.: M.C. Braude and S. Szara, Raven, New York, 1976.
8. Tashkin, D. et al. Subacute effects of heavy marijuana smoking on pulmonary function in healthy men. N.E.J. Med. 294:125-129, 1976.

8. Marijuana and Learning

Learning is a basic psychologic process. For humans learning has become a sort of external evolutionary device that supplements genetic evolutionary changes. We teach our young not only to survive, but to become civilized and sapient humans.

The society that fails to teach its young the knowledge necessary for their psychological and social development must decline. A good deal of diverse information must be acquired. This is especially true in democratic states because the citizenry must acquire a considerable data base and a decision-making capability about an ever increasing variety and complexity of issues.

Learning is, or should be, particularly rapid during the growing up period. I use the word "learning" to include not only the acquisition of factual information, but also learning how to learn and absorbing the skills needed for human growth: learning to relate to others, learning to solve problems, learning to deal with life stress, to adapt, to endure.

ESSENTIAL ELEMENTS OF LEARNING

Five elements of learning appear to dominate the educational process. The first of these is a *prepared mind*, one capable of receiving and integrating that which is to be learned. The incoming sensory information and its interdigitation with what is already known must not be distorted. The ability to sort information, discarding some and retaining other data, should not be dulled. For these purposes the sober, alert mind has been shown to be the best available instrument. No drug state can improve upon it. Although some drugs provide the illusion of mental enhancement, research has demonstrated that the undrugged brain excels for all complex mental tasks.

Another requirement is an intact *memory:* learning is not possible without the ability to remember. Recall is also necessary so that the new experience can be compared with existing stores of information.

Obviously, in order to firmly transfer and store what has been learned in the long term memory banks, *practice* is necessary. Just as learning to drive a car requires repeated driving experiences, learning to socialize, to deal with frustration, or to learn mathematics demands repetition.

As important as any factor that enters into the act of learning is *motivation*, the drive to know. Without that desire to learn, little can be learned, and an intellectual and emotional stagnation is perpetuated.

Finally, the *reinforcing or reward* aspect of acquiring new information makes a significant contribution. Learned activities tend to be perpetuated if they are rewarded. The reward may be an "A" on a report card, praise from some highly regarded person, or a self-generated feeling of satisfaction after having acquired a new skill or new information.

THE IMPACT OF MARIJUANA

Surveys have reported that marijuana is the intoxicant most likely to be used during school hours. Therefore this substance is very important to the educational system.

Intoxication with any substance is detrimental to the learning process. The sensory channels are distorted, the sorting and integrating functions develop imperfections, and remembrance is not what it should be. The "stoned" state, marijuana intoxication, although different from intoxication with alcohol or sedatives, produces aberrations in an array of mental functions that are equally impairing. It is not that no learning can occur; that will only take place at substantial degrees of intoxication. At lesser degrees something may be learned, but it might be qualitatively defective.

In addition to the learning losses that ensue during acute intoxication with marijuana, there is clinical evidence that impairment during the unintoxicated state is possible when smoking persists over months or years in the adolescent.

SENSORY AND COGNITIVE INTEGRITY AND MARIJUANA

When potent marijuana is used, the sensory changes are among the most sought-after effects. Time may slow down, and sensation is altered from an amplification (or overinterpretation) of the sensory input to illusions and, rarely, hallucinations. These alterations may be entertaining, but new learning is distorted.

Cognition varies from fanciful thinking or a reverie, dreamlike state to paranoid ideation. The ability to attend to or concentrate on the task at hand is diminished. Logical thinking may be fragmented and abstract concepts are sometimes difficult to grasp.

MEMORY AND MARIJUANA

It is well established that smoking marijuana interferes with the ability to form new memories. Immediate recall is affected by marijuana intoxication—what has just been heard, said, or done may not register. Marijuana speech exemplifies the defect. The flow of speech may come to an abrupt halt because the stoned individual cannot remember what he or she just said. This can sometimes happen to anyone (especially to elderly people), but its frequency increases under the influence of cannabis.

Impaired immediate memory leads to what Tinklenberg has called temporal disintegration, an inability to order cognitive operations that require sequential adjustments in reaching a goal.

MOTIVATION AND MARIJUANA

It is hardly surprising that acute marijuana intoxication reduces motivation and drive states. What is a cause of increasing concern to parents, educators, and physicians is the effect of long-term smoking upon adolescent motivation during periods when they are not under the influence of the drug. Adults are sometimes involved, but young people seem more vulnerable because they have not yet acquired the compensatory mechanisms for dealing with the sedation, passivity, and energy loss that accompanies chronic use.

The fullblown amotivational syndrome occurs after months or years of consistent smoking. It is readily recognized. There is a loss of ambition and initiative, a withdrawal from customary interests, and a regression to a simpler type of existence. The person is dulled, apathetic, and unconcerned, although irritable outbursts do occur when he or she is upset. Some degree of depression may be evident. Interest in schoolwork wanes and grades suffer. The youngster may drop out of school or be expelled because of absenteeism or an inability to keep up.

Lesser levels of motivational loss exist, but are not as easily identified. A decrease in energy, mild confusion, indifference, and slowness in thinking are some of the presenting manifestations.

By no means do all the heavy users of marijuana develop a loss of motivation. Many are able to compensate for the reduced drive state and continue their customary activities. Some very intelligent young people are able to get by in school even though they are functioning at a fraction of their potential. Nor should every instance of motivational loss be attributed to cannabis. Adolescent depression can present a similar picture. It is the pharmacologic effect of prolonged marijuana use, combined with a measure of psychological vulnerability that, together, result in the amotivated state caused by cannabis.

In my opinion, the condition is almost always reversible, but it can take months, even years of abstinence from marijuana for the intellectual blunting to entirely dissolve. It is interesting that, although most individuals are unaware of any mental deficit as the syndrome develops, they can recognize the "coming out of a fog" effect as it disappears.

PRACTICE AND MARIJUANA

Practice is so important to the learning process that one research psychologist (Kimble) has defined learning as: "Any long term change in behavior produced by practice." It is possible for someone to be exposed to a single learning event and never forget it. But what is more common is that we must rehearse and repeat the verbal information or behavioral skill before it becomes a part of our permanent repertoire of knowledge and behavior.

The problem with the juvenile marijuana user whose waking hours may be taken over by the "stoned" state is that even if something is learned, practice time is not available. His or her day consists of "blowing pot" after breakfast, at the 10 o'clock recess, during the lunch hour, and so on. This leaves little time for any sort of practice or review of what was learned.

REWARDS AND MARIJUANA

The problem with marijuana use during the formative years is that marijuana takes over the reward system. Marijuana becomes the major source of rewards. The incentive to learn, to study, to excel, fades because the rewards of the bedrugged state are so easily obtained. Just what incessant stimulation of the reward centers by chemicals does to the reward threshold remains unknown. If it can be compared to other neurophysiologic functions, the threshold may be raised, and ordinary pleasures may no longer be experienced as pleasurable.

DISCUSSION

How much of a public health problem are the mental and behavioral changes that can develop in the younger age groups in connection with protracted marijuana use? I can tell you of individual and family tragedies that have occurred when a child is transformed from an outgoing, achieving, friendly individual into someone withdrawn and obtunded. But how often does this happen? The casualties have not been counted, and only impressions are available. This is not an uncommon condition. Preadolescent and adolescent daily cannabis users are especially at risk. Sometimes, excessive marijuana users are also excessive alcohol users. This combination is a poor one, because both drugs impair mental functioning, although by different mechanisms. If adolescent cannabism and alcoholism are considered together, then the public health implications are serious indeed.

Most school surveys report significant decrements when scholastic achievement between nonusers and frequent users of marijuana are compared. A few do not. These latter surveys are seriously flawed on two accounts. First, they compare all marijuana users, lumping the pothead and the one-time user together and comparing them to the nonuser group. This so dilutes the chronically using groups that important differences are washed out. A second major methodological error is to ignore the dropouts from school, the very group that would contain large numbers of the most impaired cannabis smokers.

What can be done about adolescent cannabis abuse? Both the demand and the supply sides of the problem must be simultaneously engaged. Young people must be informed even though many will not listen. The parents and peer action groups are the most promising prevention programs in sight. At last the aberration called "permissiveness" has been identified, and the loving resolve to say "no" and to set limits has been relearned. A recognition of the un-drugged pleasures in life is being rediscovered. Meanwhile, supplies must be made more difficult and more expensive to obtain, and trafficking must be turned into an unrewarding enterprise.

SUMMARY

It is evident from what has been said that every element of learning is incompatible either with the acute intoxication or with the chronic mental changes that marijuana can bring. One of the most unfortunate developments of the past decade has been the increasing youth of those involved. Even elementary school teachers are becoming aware that smoking marijuana is taking place during school hours. This makes what I have said about adolescents even more ominous when applied to preteenagers.

Although the situation is somber, it is reversible. Indeed, we may be witnessing the beginnings of a turnaround now. The latest high school senior survey shows daily marijuana users at 5.5 percent, down from 10.7 percent in 1978 and 9.1 percent in 1980.

9. Cannabis: Impact on Motivation

Of all the concerns about marijuana, the public sector seems most preoccupied with its effect upon motivation, ambition, and drive states. This concern is often expressed because some parents believe they are witnessing increased passivity, disinterest, and social withdrawal in their children who indulge.

The observation is hardly a new one. It is mentioned in the first effort at an orderly evaluation of cannabis, the Indian Hemp Drugs Commission Report of 1893,[1] and by writers from many lands where potent preparations were traditionally used.[2,3,4] They noted a dull lethargy and a loss of ambition and of interest in work. These older reports have been generally disparaged by North American writers with a favorable attitude toward marijuana as inaccurate reporting by unsophisticated observers or, alternatively, due to malnutrition or worms in the indigenous population.

THE AMOTIVATIONAL SYNDROME

In 1968 two articles appeared apparently independently by McGlothlin and West[5] and by Smith[6] that used the term "amotivational syndrome" in connection with cannabis use. David Smith wrote: "Certain younger individuals who regularly use marijuana also develop what I have called the *amotivational syndrome* in that they lose the desire to work or compete." Two illustrative cases describe a lack of interest in sex, school, and other activities that remitted after a period of abstinence from cannabis.

McGlothlin and West described the syndrome as follows: "While systematic studies of the recent wave of young marijuana users are not yet available, clinical observations indicate that regular marijuana use may contribute to the development of more passive, inward turning, amotivational personality characteristics. For numerous middle class students, the progressive change from conforming, achievement-oriented behavior to a state of relaxed and careless drifting has followed their use of significant amounts of marijuana."

51

These authors believe that especially in impressionable young persons, apathy, loss of effectiveness, and diminished capacity to carry out complex long-term plans, endure frustrations, concentrate for long periods, follow routines, or successfully master new material were present. They remarked on a loss of verbal facility and of future orientation. Magical thinking, an impression of great subjective creativity but actually accompanied by a loss of productivity and withdrawal, was also mentioned.

Since then, a number of clinicians[7,8,9] and other health care professionals have provided additional reports on such adolescents and young adults who become apathetic and manifest diminished goal directedness in connection with consistent marijuana use. It seems that almost every health provider dealing with youthful clients has seen one or a series of such poorly motivated youngsters who had dropped out or who had to drop out because of an inability to keep up.

One major question that immediately arises is: Are these personality changes due to the pharmacologic action of chronic cannabis use, or are they the developmental frustrations and turmoil of certain youth who would have dropped out of the activities of living in any event?

From a review of the current available information, it appears that both possibilities occur. Some heavy smokers without pre-existing significant characterological immaturity or inadequacy have lost their previous interests and involvements. Cannabis seems to have dampened their previous level of social involvement and energy in dealing with existence. Weeks or months after discontinuing the drug they generally become more alert and can recognize their impairment in retrospect, an insight that was absent during the period of active smoking.

Another subgroup has been unable or unwilling to maintain themselves in the sometimes stressful activities associated with growing up in America and has withdrawn from active participation and engagement. For them, marijuana serves to reinforce the withdrawal and makes it more pleasant. This is not to say that the drug is incidental to the process, because re-emergence and reinvolvement in the growing up process is thereby either delayed or prevented. Therefore, writing off cannabis as merely associated with amotivation rather than causative may be incorrect if the drug substantially contributes to its perpetuation.

THEORIES OF AMOTIVATION

A number of speculations about the relationship between cannabis and amotivation is available. In no instance has any of the hypotheses listed below been proven in the scientific sense of the word.

The Cultural-Societal Theory

Those who minimize the amotivational potential of marijuana ascribe the loss of drive to the current state of societal decay in which erstwhile aspirations, beliefs, and ambitions are now untenable, even absurd. Familial, religious, and national allegiances are no longer viable, therefore there is nothing worth believing in or striving for.

Reduced to a more personal level, those in miserable living situations, or those living in more affluent situations but devoid of worthwhile and well-defined goals and ideals are obviously susceptible to disorders of motivation. The emotionally susceptible, those who do not tolerate the frustrations of daily life well, will drop out under such conditions with or without marijuana. Sometimes young people will express such sentiments as the decadence of society as a rationalization of their own inadequacies and withdrawal.

The Retained THC Theory

THC (Δ-9-tetrahydrocannabinol) with its long half-life accumulates in fat and lipid cells on repeated use. Such cumulation in the brain has been alleged to have a cytotoxic action that impairs neuronal function, disrupting complex processes like conation and motivation. This hypothesis is not proven. Evidence for THC cumulation in the brain cell has not been demonstrated.

The Louder Music and Stronger Wine Theory

It has been claimed that the incessant use of marijuana and other chemicals for pleasure eventually leads to a state that is refractory to enjoyment while in the sober condition. Sober achievements, such as active play or work no longer are a source of enjoyment and personal gratification. While this sounds like a moralistic opinion, some psychological basis for it may exist.

After prolonged exposure to altered states of consciousness one's original set of values and attitudes must change. When considerable marijuana has been used over time, motivation attenuates and shifts in the direction of regression and a diminished willingness to engage in the activities of everyday life.

The Decreased Drive Hormone Theory

Several studies have shown decreases in sex hormone levels in humans and animals. For testosterone this finding has not been invariably confirmed, and when it has been, the drop recorded is from normal to low normal levels. The reports of decreases in luteinizing hormones are more consistent. In addition to their effect on sexual drives, nonspecific drive states are also changed. The possibility that heavy users of cannabis are affected by the relative decline of circulating gonadal hormones is worth studying further.

The Brain Change Theory

Depth electrode and microscopic examinations of certain limbic system structures have revealed long-lasting changes following a six-month usage of cannabis in primates.[10] The synaptic clefts are widened and filled with radio-opaque material. The cytoplasm and the nuclei in the nerve cells involved are altered. The nerve cell endings show clumping of the storage vesicles. These changes were apparent eight months after the monkeys had stopped smoking the equivalent of three joints a day for six months. Whether this represents the neuroanatomic substrate of the amotivational syndrome is not known.

The Hemispheric Dominance Theory

Two studies have demonstrated an impairment of left hemispheric function with a subsequent relative dominance of right hemispheric activity resulting from cannabis use in some people.[11] Perhaps the repeated dampening of left hemispheric function could result in a loss of future orientation and conative behavior, but considerable additional studies are needed.

The Sedation Theory

A simple but quite probable explanation of the amotivational syndrome could be that the repeated use of any central nervous system depressant consumed during much of the waking hours can blunt responsivity and induce a loss of motivation on both an acute and a chronic basis. Persistent alcohol or sleeping pill use can certainly do this. THC has sufficient sedative activity to also produce decrements in alertness and vigor, and its cumulative property could add to the prolonged disinclination to accomplish.

The Psychic Depression Theory

The possibility that a pre-existing psychological depression or one intensified by marijuana is the cause of the amotivated state has been suggested.[14] This assumption is tenable for certain individuals involved with marijuana but does not explain most other instances.

ARGUMENTS AGAINST THE AMOTIVATIONAL SYNDROME

Some school surveys of marijuana vs. nonmarijuana users have shown no particular difference in achievement or performance between the two groups.[12,13] In general, such survey results suffer from two deficiencies. The amount of marijuana smoked was less than the quantities smoked at present. Even a few years ago "heavy users" were often defined as those who smoked only three or more times a week. A second problem with such studies was that dropouts from school were not included in the study. Thus, a crucial indicator of amotivation may have been excluded.

Perhaps the best evidence that cannabis does not induce amotivation comes from naturalistic studies done during the past 10 years in Jamaica, Costa Rica, and Greece. The Jamaican study[15] consisted of 30 cannabis users selected from a much larger group, and 30 controls matched for age, residence, and socioeconomic status.

Ganja (marijuana) is considered to be an energizer among Jamaican laborers and farmers. Owners make it available to farm hands because they are believed to work harder under its influence. Ganja breaks are taken, analogous to the coffee breaks in North America.

An increased social cohesiveness during work was noted, and negative effects of ganja smoking upon the work output were not obtained. When light, moderate, and heavy smokers were videotaped and studied, the heavy smokers were found to work longer, but to expend more energy at any given task. No gross defect in intellectual abilities was found when the smokers were compared with the control group.

The Costa Rican sample consisted of 41 cannabis users and a like number of controls matched for age, mental status, education, occupation, and alcohol and tobacco consumption. The authors[16] concluded that cannabis is not an amotivator. This opinion was based upon the finding that the onset of age of regular work was the same for both groups. There was also no dose relationship among the users with respect to occupational achievement or social adjustment. The heaviest users were more successful than those who smoked lesser amounts.

It was evident, however, from the data provided, that users did change jobs more frequently, had jobs that were part-time or temporary, and had longer unemployment periods.

They had fewer pay raises and promotions and were more likely to indulge in extralegal activities than the controls. From the information given it is difficult to completely agree with the conclusion that cannabis did not impair the ganja group. In addition, important differences in socialization existed between the two groups as manifested by the number of school problems and in delinquent activities.

For example, 36 percent of the users were sentenced to a reformatory in contrast to none of the controls, and the arrests were not for offenses in connection with cannabis. Eighty-three percent of users received sentences for delinquent acts compared with none of the controls. The authors suggest these high arrest and sentencing rates were caused by the labelling of marijuana smokers and their selective arrest by the authorities.

The authors also wondered if the users became involved in marijuana during their reformatory stay. This is unlikely since the paper points out that they started smoking as children and were regular consumers by the onset of adolescence. The large number of arrests and convictions by users cannot be summarily written off as police harassment of ganja users when we read that delinquent activities were more common among the users shortly after smoking began.

It may be concluded from the article that not everyone becomes amotivated as a result of substantial cannabis consumption. However, a subgroup does seem to be affected, and their subsequent life-styles are influenced by continuing ganja use.

Two groups of heavy hashish Greek users, one with 40 and another with 30 subjects along with a like number of controls, were studied. These were illiterate or semiliterate individuals. No significant differences in mood, thought, and behavior were detected. The cannabis group had higher rates both for unemployment and for arrests even when arrests for marijuana were not included.[17]

A POSSIBLE EXPLANATION OF THE NEGATIVE FINDINGS

An Egyptian study may help clarify some of the issues raised by the Greek, Costa Rican, and Jamaican investigations.

A total of 1,054 hashish users was compared with 954 controls, all imprisoned in Cairo or in rural jails.[18] A battery of culture-appropriate tests of intelligence and other aspects of mental functioning was administered.

It was found that the illiterate, the rural, and the older subgroups tended to have smaller test score deficits when the hashish and control groups were compared. Increased literacy, urban residence, and youthfulness were factors associated with markedly lower scores in the cannabis users vs. the controls on 10 of the 16 tests. These results may explain the nonsignificant difference between users and nonusers in the Costa Rican, Greek, and Jamaican studies, since their subjects were all unskilled laborers, farmers, or urban ghetto dwellers.

Apparently chronic cannabis use does not—or cannot—reduce motivation and intellectual activity in populations with pre-existing low intellectual skills or nonstimulating life styles. It will impair those who live in a complicated society that demands precision thinking to achieve and survive. The increased impact of cannabis consumption on youth as contrasted with older users is also of interest since similar conclusions were reached on the basis of clinical impressions reported from North America and Western Europe.

Another possible explanation of the differences in various studies reporting on the phenomenon was suggested by Petersen.[19] The customary manner of smoking cannabis in this country is the deep inhalation and the retention of the smoke in the lungs as long as possible. The technique increases the efficiency of the extraction of THC. In Jamaica where the cannabis is mixed with tobacco, the smoking procedure resembles cigar smoking more, with little or no deep inhalation, and therefore with less absorption of the cannabinoids.

There is another reason why the tests performed on laborers and farmers may not be applicable to those who are involved in complex life styles. Boring work may, indeed, be done as well or better under the intoxicating influence of cannabis. From what we know of cannabis' effects on memory, perception, cognition, and the integration of complex mental processes, it is evident that complicated work that includes the processing of new information is performed with greater difficulty.

The Canadian commission[20] as a result of its own contracted study concluded that cannabis can, in certain circumstances, reduce motivation for performing some tasks. It pointed out that similar effects occur with alcohol use. In students they found that the greater the use of cannabis, the greater the decline in grades.

Heavy users had higher failure rates than light or nonusers. A drop in final grade averages was noted in 77 percent of heavy users. Impaired abstracting and synthesizing of information, and difficulty in grasping the appropriateness of their behavior led to motivational change and apathy. The unanswered question was: Is the change due to heavy cannabis use or to participation in a culture that did not want academic success or did not value activities such as planning, concern for the future, or rationality?

The 1979 National Survey on Drug Abuse[21] obtained opinions on favorable and unfavorable effects of marijuana use from the respondents. An inquiry on the amotivational syndrome (operationally defined as: "Would make a hardworking person stop caring and not try as hard") was made of young adults (18–25) and older adults (25+). Of the young adults, most of whom (68 percent) had smoked marijuana, 40 percent believed that smoking every night and on weekends to stay high would decrease motivation.

If marijuana were smoked every day and at night so that one was almost always high, then 65 percent assumed that motivation would be impaired. Among the older adults (20 percent had used marijuana) 61 percent believed that night and weekend smoking would diminish motivation and 78 percent believed that being almost always high would diminish motivation.

Kolansky and Moore[8] collected 51 patients who developed undesired effects from cannabis that correlated well with the duration and frequency of smoking. Early psychiatric changes included a diminution of self-awareness and judgment. Later, slowed thinking and diminished concentration and attention span appeared. Eventually, lack of goals, blunting of emotions, and a sort of counterfeit calm overlaid the mental impairment. These were accompanied by illusions of insight and emotional maturity.

Kupfer et al.[14] studied three groups of patients. Forty-four had smoked marijuana up to twice a week and were considered light smokers. Forty-six had used marijuana three or more times a week and were called heavy smokers. The comparison group was made up of nonsmoking patients with some psychiatric diagnosis. All were given tests of personality, behavior, and mood.

Those in the heavily smoking group were found to be more anxious and fatigued and had difficulties in relating to people. They were also significantly more depressed or had organic brain dysfunction on testing than the light smokers, and their levels of depression and organicity approached that of the psychiatric patient group. This study confirms others insofar as the mood and cognitive changes of heavy smokers are concerned. On the other hand it is possible that a self-selection process was involved, with the psychologically sicker people tending to use marijuana more heavily.

Mellinger et al.[22] have provided a series of papers indicating that the inability to stay in college, get good grades, and define occupational goals is affected by marijuana and other drug use. Whether high levels of marijuana use produces low academic motivation, or whether low academic motivation induces marijuana use is sometimes difficult to sort out. At any rate the chronic user is unlikely to have ordinary levels of motivation and the infrequent user is not likely to be impaired. The authors stress that nondrug factors such as educational background, family relationships, and academic indecision are important variables in the dropping-out process.

DISCUSSION

Since motivation or the lack of it is difficult to define operationally, research studies are difficult to design. Animal models of sustained amotivation do not, of course, exist. Human experimentation, that is, deliberately giving large amounts of marijuana for long periods in a naturalistic setting to examine motivational levels, is ethically unjustifiable.

Prospective studies, in which sufficiently large groups of young people are followed for years and their marijuana careers and their school and job achievements are evaluated, are possible but expensive and not easily executed. Apparently, such studies have not yet been started.

It is necessary to separate the decreased drive associated with the acute intoxicated state from motivational loss during the interim—while not using cannabis—in the chronic smoker. It would be anticipated that any kind of acute depressant drug intoxication will decrease motivation. In fact acute cannabis intoxication clearly impairs intellectual performance on a wide range of mental functions.[23]

Complex reaction time, immediate recall, concept formation, reading comprehension, speech, and other cognitive tasks all have consistently been adversely affected. What is more important insofar as motivation is concerned, is whether or not the residual effects of the drug continue to diminish the desire or ability to function over protracted periods—what is called burnout by those in contact with such individuals.

It is not unlikely that simple, repetitive tasks are performed as well by poorly motivated individuals as by others. Skilled activities requiring judgments and decision making on the other hand, are less likely to be adequately performed while acutely stoned or chronically blunted.

Whether marijuana is a primary or secondary factor in inducing amotivation is not a crucial issue. A drug that simply served, in certain instances, to support and reinforce passivity and withdrawal, would make it an undesirable agent for predisposed individuals.

The possibility that psychologically and chronologically immature individuals are more likely to be involved in loss of motivation is an important point. Clinical impressions amply support this view. It is not necessary to invoke altered metabolic pathways in young vs. old people. Instead, it is more likely that the immature of all ages, and certainly those with low initial levels of motivation, are more likely to be overwhelmed by the euphoro-sedative effects of cannabis.[24]

REFERENCES

1. *Indian Hemp Drugs Commission Report 1893-1894*. Silver Springs, Md., Thomas Jefferson Pub., reprinted 1969, p. 3281.
2. Benabud, A. Psychopathological aspects of the cannabis situation in Morocco. Statistical data for 1956. U.N. Bull. Narcotics. 9:1–16, 1957.
3. Miras, C. J. *Drugs and Youth*. Springfield; C. C. Thomas, 1969.
4. Chopra, I.C. and Chopra, R.N. The use of the cannabis drugs in India. U.N. Bull. Narcotics. 9:4–29, 1957.
5. McGlothlin, W. H. and West, L. J. The marijuana problem: An overview. Amer. J. Psychiat. 125:1126–1134, 1968.
6. Smith, D. E. The acute and chronic toxicity of marijuana. J. Psychedelic Drugs. 2:(2)37–48, 1968.
7. Sharma, B. P. Cannabis and its users in Nepal. Brit. J. Psychol. 127: 550–552, 1975.
8. Kolansky, H. and Moore, W. T. Total effects of marijuana use. J.A.M.A. 222:35–41, 1972.

9. Campbell, I. The amotivational syndrome and cannabis use with emphasis on the Canadian scene. Ann. N.Y. Acad. Sci. 282: 33–36, 1976.
10. Heath, R. G. Cannabis sativa derivatives: Effects on brain function in monkeys. In G. G. Nahas (Ed.) *Marijuana: Chemistry, Biochemistry and Cellular Effects*. Springer Verlag, New York, 1976.
11. Harshman, R. A., Crawford, H. J. and Hecht, E. Marijuana cognitive style and lateralized hemispheric functions. In: S. Cohen and R. S. Stillman (Eds.) *The Therapeutic Potential of Marijuana*. Plenum, New York, 1976.
12. Hogan, R. et al. Personality correlates of undergraduate marijuana use. J. Consult. Clin. Psychol. 35: 58–63, 1970.
13. Brill, N. Q. and Christie, R. L. Marijuana use and psycho-social adaptation. Arch. Gen. Psychiat. 31:713–719, 1974.
14. Kupfer, D. J. et al. A comment on the amotivational syndrome in marijuana smokers. Amer. J. Psychiat. 130: 1319–1322, 1973.
15. Comitas, L. Cannabis and work in Jamaica. A refutation of the amotivational hypothesis. Ann. N.Y. Acad. Sci. 282: 24-32, 1976.
16. Carter, W.E. and Doughty, P.L. Social and cultural aspects of cannabis use in Costa Rica. Ann. N.Y. Acad. Sci. 282: 2-16, 1976.
17. Boulougouris, J. C., Liakos, A. and Stepanis, C. Social traits of heavy hashish users and matched controls. Ann. N.Y. Acad. Sci. 282:17–23, 1976.
18. Soueif, M. I. Differential association between chronic cannabis use and brain function deficits. Ann. N.Y. Acad. Sci. 282: 323–343, 1976.
19. Petersen, R. C. Importance of inhalation patterns in determining effects of marijuana use. Lancet 1:727–728 (Mar. 30), 1979.
20. *Cannabis: A Report of the Commission of Inquiry into the Non-medical Use of Drugs*. Catalogue No. H 21–530/4, Information Canada, Ottawa, 1972.
21. Miller, J. D. and Cisin, I. H. *Highlights from the National Survey on Drug Abuse: 1979*. NIDA, 5600 Fishers Lane, Rockville, Md. 20857.
22. Mellinger, G. D. et al. The amotivational syndrome and the college student. Ann. N.Y. Acad. Sci. 282: 37–55, 1976.
23. NIDA Research Monograph #31. *Marijuana Research Findings 1980*. Ed. R. C. Petersen, U.S. Government Printing Office, Washington, D.C. 20402, 1980.
24. *Marijuana and Youth: Clinical Observations on Motivation and Learning*. DHHS Publication No. (ADM) 82–1186. U.S. Government Printing Office, Washington, D.C. 20402, 1982.

10. Marijuana and the Public Health: An Analysis of Four Major Reports

During the past 3 years four important reports on cannabis from national and international scientific bodies have been issued. These are worth reviewing since public information lags behind the latest clinical and research findings, and significant new data are at hand.

Three of the reports will be considered together because they are generally in agreement, although differences in emphasis exist. These are from the National Institute of Drug Abuse (NIDA), the Institute of Medicine (IOM), and the World Health Organization (WHO). A fourth document from the National Research Council (NRC) will be analyzed separately.

GENERAL CONCLUSIONS

The NIDA[2] summary noted the limited amount of research information available, especially on long-term effects. The American pattern of usage: widespread, sometimes intensive, use by adolescents of both sexes in a demanding, industrialized society, is unprecedented. The historical pattern of initial optimism that follows the discovery or rediscovery of a pleasure-giving drug eventually gives way to an awareness of enduringly high personal and societal costs. Marijuana is unlikely to be an exception. It is disquieting to note that marijuana is at least five times more potent than it was five years ago and that the age of onset of usage is declining. Although the number of high school seniors who use the drug daily has decreased to 5.5 percent (from 10.7 percent in 1978), it still is the most frequently used daily drug. Alcohol is used by 5 percent daily.

The overall IOM[1] conclusion is worth quoting. "What little we know about the effects of marijuana on human health—and all we have reason to suspect—justifies serious national concern."

The WHO[3] summary states that "intermittent use of low potency cannabis is not generally associated with obvious symptoms of toxicity. Daily or more frequent use, especially of the highly potent preparations, can produce a chronic intoxication which may take several weeks to clear after drug use is discontinued."

SPECIFIC EFFECTS

The Mind and Behavior

All three reviews agree on the negative impact of the acute intoxicated state for overall mental functioning, classroom performance, driving, and related complex tasks. The effect on learning is pertinent, since much marijuana use occurs during school hours. The psychomotor deficits can last up to 4 to 10 hours after smoking, well beyond the duration of "high."

In the area of chronic mental effects from persistent smoking, additional research is urgently needed. The demonstration of microscopic alterations on monkeys' brain structures for example, requires replication. The three reports pay particular attention to the issue of loss of motivation due to cannabis. The IOM statement is representative. "The possible role of marijuana in causing an amotivational syndrome is a matter of great concern. Apathy, poor school or work performance, and lack of goals characterize a number of long-term users. But it has not been possible to know how much was caused by use of marijuana and how much was antecedent; it seems likely that both factors (drug effects and self-selection) contribute to the motivational problems seen in chronic users of marijuana. Existing studies have produced conflicting results. None of the investigators have looked at effects on the very young daily marijuana user who is regarded as potentially at high risk for damaging effects because of physiological and psychological immaturity."

The NIDA position includes a reliance on clinical findings. It states: "There are disturbing clinical reports of behavioral disruption and loss of conventional motivation related to marijuana use. In addition, a significant percentage of daily users in nationwide surveys report the presence of components of the amotivational syndrome."

The WHO statement reminds us that the persistence of THC metabolites in body fat may indicate a continuing interference with body functions, but definite evidence is lacking. It notes that the finding of impaired short-term memory is because of marijuana's interference with the acquisition and storage of new data. The IOM report points out that interactions with alcohol can increase the mental changes. Adolescents and the elderly may be more sensitive to the effects of cannabis. People with mental illness might be made worse.

Agreement is unanimous with regard to impairment of driving performance. Alone or combined with alcohol, it has been implicated in traffic accidents and fatalities. The driving skill disruption is dose related. Safe driving is impaired by decrements in coordination, tracking, perception, recognition, immediate recall, cognition, time sense, and learning. Tests in driving simulators, test automobile courses under actual traffic conditions, and information derived from accident surveys all show impairment following the use of ordinary amounts of marijuana.

Effects on the Lungs

The three reports agree that marijuana contains carcinogenic chemicals. Marijuana tars contain 50 percent more carcinogens than high-tar tobacco cigarettes, with 70 percent more benzopyrene in marijuana than in tobacco smoke (WHO). Marijuana smoke is mutagenic (causes genetic changes in 4 of 5 bacterial strains) (IOM). When bits of lung tissue were exposed to marijuana smoke, striking changes were seen. When recent hashish smokers were biopsied, their lung microstructure resembled that of chronic heavy tobacco smokers including atypical cells and basal cell hyperplasia (precancerous lesions). There was general agreement that the combined use of marijuana and tobacco was worse than either substance alone. Rodent skins painted with marijuana tars developed tumors just as with tobacco tars. The WHO recommendation was that marijuana smokers should be monitored for lung cancer development. At this time direct confirmation of the generation of human lung cancers by marijuana is not yet at hand (NIDA).

After an initial bronchodilation, chronic smoking leads to a mild but significant large airway resistance. In hashish users rhinitis, sinusitis, pharyngitis, and bronchitis were noted (WHO). Although impaired macrophage (large cells in the lung that take up bacteria and other foreign bodies) activity has been reported, it is not conclusively confirmed (IOM).

Effects on the Heart

The most obvious effect of marijuana on the heart is a brisk increase in heart rate, an increase that can reach 160 beats per minute in some instances (WHO). Although not threatening to the normal heart, except during maximal exercise, this can be harmful to the failing heart or one with coronary artery narrowing. A sudden drop in blood pressure on arising can cause faintness in some people.

Effects on the Reproductive Systems

The consensus is that the human research is incomplete. The animal work shows a consistent toxicity at doses comparable to those consumed by daily users. In a variety of species gonadotropins (hormones that control reproductive function), testosterone and leutinizing hormone levels are lowered. Ovulation (egg maturation) is compromised and sperm production is diminished.

Other Effects

Chromosomal changes have been described, but the research requires further confirmation. Studies of immune response in the human are contradictory. The effect should be established by further work because of the important implications of even a mild impairment of immunoreactivity. The clinical significance of the DNA and RNA inhibition found in cells exposed to marijuana smoke cannot be established at this time. The IOM report suggests that promising findings have been mentioned when the drug is used for certain therapeutic indications, and that research should continue.

RECOMMENDATIONS OF THE THREE REPORTS

Further investigations are needed in specific areas particularly in adolescents and other vulnerable populations. The list of high risk populations is similar to that mentioned in *The Substance Abuse Problems*, Vol. I, p. 39.

THE NATIONAL RESEARCH COUNCIL (NRC) REPORT[4]

General Conditions

This report recognizes that "concern with the health hazards attributable to marijuana have been rising and are not to be taken lightly. Heavy use by anyone or any use by children should be discouraged. The likelihood of developmental damage to some young users makes marijuana use a cause for extreme concern."

Despite this, the effectiveness of complete prohibition has failed to prevent use. The policy of partial prohibition (prohibition of supplies such as trafficking and transporting for sale) is recommended because of lower costs. Even controlling supplies has been demonstrated to be ineffective. "Hence a variety of alternative policies should be considered." Regulation (legalization) is one option that should be studied.

Comment

The NRC paper is remarkable in a number of respects.

1. The President of the National Academy of Sciences (NAS), Frank Press, felt compelled to publicly disagree with the recommendations of a NAS

report. (The NRC is the research arm of the NAS.) He writes in a letter of transmittal of the NRC report: "My own view is that the data available to the (NRC) Committee were insufficient to justify on scientific or analytical grounds changes in current policies dealing with the use of marijuana." It is most unusual for an NAS President to disagree with a report coming from his own organization. Press points out further: "I fear that this report coming as it does from a well-known and well-respected scientific organization will be misunderstood by the media and the public to imply that new scientific data are suddenly available that justify sudden changes in public attitudes on the use of marijuana."

2. Other grounds for criticism exist beyond those mentioned by Frank Press. The NRC Committee seemed to have relied heavily upon *Marijuana: A Signal of Misunderstanding*,[5] a document written by a National Commission 11 years ago and obsolescent in view of the research data that have emerged since.

3. The NRC group placed great weight on the point that no increase in the numbers or the intensity of marijuana use has occurred in those states that decriminalized the drug. In fact, no scientifically acceptable study has been done on this point.

4. Throughout the report selective citations, selective in support of its conclusions, were used. Just as valid and available contrary views were not presented.

5. The claim is made that a college student survey by Hochman and Brill (done 10 years ago) has tempered earlier fears of an amotivational syndrome. Actually, that issue is more alive today than ever, and is established from a clinical standpoint.

6. The membership of the NRC Committee is first-rate. This makes some of their evaluations and judgments difficult to understand.

7. The report reveals an innocence about the marijuana street scene. During its ruminations about legalization and the placing of limits on the potency of marijuana, it mentions that such limits might still result in a substantial hashish black market. A glance at the percentages of THC in confiscated marijuana would have apprised the Committee that marijuana is now as strong as hashish in THC content.

8. The Committee perpetuates the not quite logical notion that since alcohol and tobacco are health hazards, therefore regulating (legalizing) marijuana

is proper. In effect, what they are saying is: since we have two health hazards, why not add a third?

9. A statement without any basis whatsoever is: "If many dealers who sell cocaine, PCP, amphetamines, and barbiturates as well as marijuana would be put out of business if marijuana were made available through legal channels, it might result in a curtailed market for a variety of other drugs." It is even more likely that the opposite would happen, and dealers would push their other items even more.

Why has the Committee come to its conclusions without adequate deliberation or scientific rigor? Perhaps it was because too few of the members were expert in the biologic and clinical aspects of cannabis. Another possibility is that a "committee persuasion" phenomenon produced this poorly thought through report. It has been well demonstrated that when one or a very small number of committee members are strongly for or against a report, the small but vigorous minority's position will prevail. This is what may have happened to the NRC report.

SUMMARY

All four reports agree that to consider marijuana a harmless drug is untenable. The NRC policy statement is flawed on many points, probably because it is a decade out-of-date.

REFERENCES

1. Institute of Medicine. Marijuana and Health. National Academy Press, Washington, D.C., 1982.
2. National Institute on Drug Abuse. Marijuana and Health: Ninth Report to the U.S. Congress. DHHS Publ. No. 82–1216, Washington, D.C., 1982.
3. World Health Organization. Report of an ARF/WHO Scientific Meeting on Adverse Consequences of Cannabis Use. Addiction Research Foundation, Toronto, 1981.
4. National Research Council. An Analysis of Marijuana Policy. National Academy Press, 2101 Constitution Ave., N.W., Washington, D.C., 20418, 1982.
5. National Commission on Marijuana and Drug Abuse. Marijuana: A Signal of Misunderstanding. U.S. Government Printing Office, Washington, D.C., 1972.

11. Marijuana and Reproductive Functions

The effects of cannabis upon the reproductive system are not easily reviewed because the system itself is a complicated one with considerable diurnal and lunar variations. The research is far from complete, and it suffers from contradictory reports, unreplicated findings, and heterogeneous methodology. However, a considerable amount of fairly reliable information is now available, and a few definite statements applicable to the human situation can be made.

We have the advantage of an excellent animal model for human reproduction. In fact, much of the physiology and neuroanatomy, the multiple neurohormonal interactions, the releasing hormones, and the rhythmic target organ endocrine surges are derived from it. The model is the rhesus monkey, a primate that provides an excellent facsimile of human reproductive function, with the female cyclings similar to those of the human primate.

A summary of the various animal and human studies will be provided with the disclaimer that revisions may have to be made in years to come.

MALE SEXUAL EFFECTS

Testicular Function

A number of reports have shown that cannabis and THC lower testosterone levels in male rodents. The Leydig cells, producers of that hormone, have been observed to be impaired in mice provided with marijuana. Leutinizing hormone (LH) was reduced in these studies. Plasma testosterone levels in primates are variable with some investigations noting decreases and a few mentioning no change following marijuana smoking.

Assuming that a decrease occurs, the significance of the decrease remains doubtful. In our study,[1] for example, the mean drop on days when marijuana was not used went from 733ng/100ml to 716ng/100ml after 180 minutes. On those days when a single 900mg, 2 percent marijuana cigarette was smoked by the same subjects, the plasma testosterone dropped from 779ng/100ml before smoking to 505ng/100ml 180 minutes later. The range of normal values for the method used was 380 to 980ng/100ml. The question becomes; is a low normal value clinically meaningful compared to a high normal value? Possibly during puberty, when marked alterations of sexual development are taking place, a slight change in testosterone concentration could impact on biobehavioral maturation.

LH is suppressed in most species, but follicle stimulating hormone seems to be unchanged following acute marijuana use.

Several levels of gonadal hormonal control are possible: (1) Neurotransmitters to the hypothalamus like dopamine and serotonin modulate secretion of (2) gonadotropin releasing hormone which increases the discharge of (3) pituitary gonadotropins into the circulation which (4) increases the production of LH and testosterone in the testicles. The cannabis effect is presumed to be at the hypothalamic centers, but evidence for higher and lower involvement also exists.

Testicular Structure

THC and marijuana produce a loss of weight of rat reproductive organs. This change is reversible on discontinuing chronic usage. Interference with sperm maturation and seminiferous tubule degeneration in rats have been reported.[2] Mice show an increase in the number of abnormal sperm. It has been assumed that cannabinoids inhibit protein synthesis in the gonads accounting for the aberrant sperm forms. One study found a decrease in fertility, not only in the adult male mice given cannabinoids, but also in their untreated male offspring.[3] Heavy marijuana smoking in men resulted in decreased numbers and concentration of sperm. The number and motility of normal sperm were reduced.[8]

FEMALE REPRODUCTIVE EFFECTS

Ovarian Function

A number of studies report temporary reductions in LH and prolactin in female rodents given single doses of THC. Follicle-stimulating hormone was not affected. One report mentioned a marked postnatal mortality among rat pups from mothers given THC. These deaths were apparently due to failure of lactation because cross-fostering of pups by the control mothers resulted in their survival, whereas pups from control mothers fostered by THC-dosed mothers had an increased mortality.

The long-term exposure of female rhesus monkeys to injections of THC caused disruptions of the menstrual cycles. For months ovulation ceased and gonadotropin and estrogen levels were reduced. Despite continued administration of THC over a half year, normal cycles were re-established. It appears that tolerance to the ovulatory and menstrual distortions occurs.[4] The observation is analogous to another study which found that regular users of marijuana experienced a similar development of tolerance. They noticed menstrual distortions initially, but as they continued to smoke, normal cycles resumed.

The search for the site of action of THC continues. As with males, suppression of LH secretion may originate in the changed cerebral neurotransmitter pattern, the hypothalamic gonadotrophic releasing hormones, the pituitary reproductive hormones, or a direct action on ovarian estrogens, or combinations of these. The contribution of a direct effect upon the ovary requires brief elaboration. THC concentrates in the corpus luteum of mice because of its lipophillic propensity. It has also been found that the ovarian follicles of THC-treated rodents contain lower amounts of prostaglandin E which could interfere with the rhythm of ovulation.

Human females who had used marijuana four times a week or more were compared with women who had never used the drug. It was found that marijuana-using women had significantly shorter cycles, a consequence of shorter luteal phases. Prolactin levels were significantly lower, and testosterone concentrations significantly higher. The elevation of testosterone in females and its possible lowering in males are not necessarily inconsistent. In men testosterone is produced in the testes, in women it is manufactured in the adrenal cortex.

Some preliminary findings from another study reported that galactorrhea occurred in 20 percent of the marijuana-using group, a figure which seems high for a normal group of women.[5]

Ovarian Structure

The chronic administration of THC in mice at a dose comparable to daily human smokers induced a significant increase in abnormal ova. The mice were at an age corresponding to the prepubertal stage of human sexual maturation. Although the percentage of abnormal ova was only 5.5 percent above the control group, the biological significance could be important. New ova are not generated after birth, and an increase in defective ova of that magnitude could significantly affect the number of fetal deaths or abnormalities over the reproductive life of a woman.

Pregnancy

Animal studies and retrospective examinations of women who have used marijuana regularly during pregnancy indicate that stillbirths and neonatal deaths are increased. Precipitate labor and meconium passage were more frequent in human marijuana users than in a control group.[6]

While looking for growth and physical anomalies related to the fetal alcohol syndrome, a group at Boston City Hospital[7] found that marijuana made more of a contribution to birth-weight decreases than alcohol. Cigarette smoking had an even greater effect than the other two drugs. A second study in Denver replicated these findings. Insofar as fetal anomalies were concerned, marijuana users were five times more likely than nonusers to deliver a child with features of the fetal alcohol syndrome.[7] Another clinical study confirmed these findings. In taking history from mothers of six infants with the fetal alcohol syndrome, all the mothers denied use of alcohol during pregnancy but admitted cigarette and marijuana smoking, the latter from two to 14 times daily.[7] It appears that both alcohol and cannabis can produce what is called the fetal alcohol syndrome.

Tremors and a high-pitched cry were noted in newborns whose mothers used marijuana daily. The relationship remained significant when nicotine and alcohol were partialed out. These changes disappeared in one month.

Marijuana is used during pregnancy by a sufficient number of women to represent a health hazard. The reported use by pregnant females varies between 10 and 37 percent and is comparable to the 26 percent of marijuana-using women between the ages of 18 and 25. The preliminary studies cited above must be replicated before definite statements can be made. Confounding the problem is the fact that marijuana may be part of a polydrug syndrome.

Like other unnecessary drugs, marijuana should not be used during pregnancy. While the data on low birth weight and fetal abnormalities are only suggestive, it is always prudent to avoid a possible embryotoxin.

THC is transferred across the placenta and into maternal milk. Its use should be avoided during the period of nursing. The marijuana-using mother's motivation to give maternal care requires investigation.

Unfortunately, marijuana is sometimes consumed with tobacco and alcohol, drugs which have a reputation for producing low neonatal weight and deforming congenital changes. The combined use of the three substances can be assumed to be worse for the fetus than either drug alone.

REFERENCES

1. Kolodny, R.C. et al. Depression of plasma testosterone with acute marijuana administration. In: *Pharmacology of Marijuana*, Eds.: M.C. Braude and S. Szara. Raven Press, New York, 1981, pp. 217–225.
2. Rosencrantz, H. and Hayden, D.W. Acute and subacute inhalation tox-

icity of Turkish marijuana, cannabochromene and cannobidiol in rats. Toxicol. Appl. Pharmacol. 28:18–27, 1974.

3. Dalterio, S. et al. Cannabinoids in male mice. Effects on fertility and spermatogenesis. Science 216:315–316, 1982.

4. Smith, C.G. et al. Tolerance develops to the disruptive effects of Δ9 THC on primate menstrual cycle. Science 219:1453–1455, 1983.

5. Mendelson, J.H. and Mello, N.K. Effect of marijuana on neuroendocrine hormones in human males and females. In: *Marijuana Effects on the Endocrine and Reproductive Systems*. Eds.: M.C. Braude and J.P. Ludford. NIDA Research Monograph 44. National Institute on Drug Abuse, 5600 Fishers Lane, Rockville, MD 20857, 1984, pp. 97–114.

6. Tennes, K. Effects of marijuana on pregnancy and fetal development in the human. In: *Marijuana Effects on the Endocrine and Reproductive Systems*. Eds.: M.C. Braude and J.P. Ludford. NIDA Research Monograph 44, National Institute on Drug Abuse, 5600 Fishers Lane, Rockville, MD 20857, pp. 115–124, 1984.

7. Hingston, R. et al. Effects of maternal drinking and marijuana use on fetal growth and development. Pediatrics 70: 539–546, 1982.

8. Hembree, W.C. et al. Changes in human spermatozoa associated with high dose marijuana smoking. In: *Marijuana: Biological Effects*. Eds.: G.G. Nahas and W.D.M. Patton, Pergamon Press, Oxford, 1979.

12. Cancer Chemotherapy and Vomiting: THC and Other Antiemetics

This chapter was written by Sidney Cohen, M.D., and Therese Andrysiak, R.N. Ms. Andrysiak has been coordinator of marijuana research at the Neuropsychiatric Institute, UCLA.

The nausea and vomiting associated with cancer chemotherapy are serious limiting factors that can interfere with the treatment program. Patients can become depleted from the loss of fluids, electrolytes, and nutrients. Anorexia prevents adequate caloric intake, and considerable weight loss and exhaustion occur. Because of the severity of the adverse effects, patients have been known to refuse further chemotherapy and seek out alternative, sometimes dubious, treatments. In a few instances the gastrointestinal distress has led physicians to cancel or reduce the planned dosage below optimal levels. Extreme retching has been reported to result in esophageal tears and rib fractures. It is surprising that, until recently, research into the causes and management of the emetic effects of the anticancer agents has not been more vigorously investigated.

THE NATURE OF VOMITING

Nausea, vomiting, and retching can be induced by noxious stimuli from receptor areas in the periphery, the cerebral cortex, the chemoreceptor trigger zones, or from combinations of these. Irritation of the pharynx, the stomach, or the inner ear exemplify peripheral vomiting stimuli. Cisplatin is an especially emetic anticancer drug, and it appears to act primarily on the gastrointestinal tract with transmission via the vagus to the emetic center in the medulla.[1]

The central or cortical pathways can instigate emesis from disgusting sights or nauseating thoughts, and these may be mediated by dopaminergic

neurons to the emetic center. The phenomenon of anticipatory vomiting origi-
nates in the cortex. Nesse et al.[2] consider this a conditioned response to the
effects of the treatment. The patient has heard that cancer chemotherapeutic
agents can cause vomiting, or has experienced such disagreeable symptoms
during previous courses. On the day that the treatment is scheduled, the patient becomes nauseated and vomits before receiving the chemotherapy.

Many of the agents used to treat cancer act over the chemoreceptor trigger
zone (CTZ) in the medulla on the floor of the fourth ventricle. This area responds to circulating chemicals in the blood stream. 5-flourouracil is an anticancer compound that causes vomiting by stimulating of the CTZ.

Distinct from the CTZ is the emetic center, the effector site that coordi-
nates the complex act of vomiting: breath holding, diaphragmatic spasm, anti-
peristalsis, salivation, and contraction of the abdominal muscles. The emetic
center receives impulses from the periphery, the higher brain centers, and the
CTZ, and it orchestrates the act of vomiting. The emetic center is not directly
affected by the anticancer drugs.

IS IT ALL IN ONE'S HEAD?

Chang[3] believes that much of the nausea and vomiting experienced by cancer patients undergoing chemotherapy is central in origin. He makes the following points:

1. These patients have an unresolved fear of death, with those who have
emotionally accepted their poor prognosis suffering less with vomiting.

2. Children, mentally retarded persons, and others with a lowered awareness of the seriousness of their illness seem to be less troubled with vomiting.

3. Angry, anxious, or skeptical patients are more likely to have severe
gastric emesis.

4. Antiemetics like Compazine, Haldol, metaclopramide, and THC are
sedative, and this may be related to their antiemetic efficacy.

5. Placebos are effective in about a quarter of chemotherapy patients.

6. Psychotherapy and support of the patient can be effective.

7. The anticipatory vomiting mentioned above is another indication of the
central origin of the vomiting.

It is obvious that input from the cerebral cortex can modulate the vomiting center. However, the notion that the nausea and vomiting that accompany cancer chemotherapy are entirely psychological does not satisfy all the known facts.

1. Test animals given the emesis-inducing cancer drugs will vomit.

2. Roentgen irradiation causes nausea and vomiting only when the treatment is directed at the trunk. Malignancies treated in other areas are associated with little or no emesis.

3. Stronger sedatives (barbiturates, for example) than the antiemetic drugs are effective only at hypnotic doses.

4. The efficacy of the antiemetic drugs does not correlate well with their sedative effect.

5. Certain anticancer drugs do not produce vomiting (vincristine, for example). If the idea that emesis is caused by the emotional disturbance associated with cancer is true, then all anticancer drugs should induce the condition.

THE ANTIEMETICS

1. Compazine and other *phenothiazines* (Torecan, Thorazine) are the standard antiemetics. They appear to act at the level of the CTZ and block the transmission of dopamine-containing neurones. Although superior to a placebo, they are effective in only about half of the symptomatic patients.

2. As might be expected, Haldol and droperidol also act in the CTZ and also block dopaminergic transmission. These *butyrophenones* may be more effective against the strong emetics like cisplatin, mechlorethamine, and doxorubicin, but this has not been proven with controlled studies. Domperidone, not yet available in this country, appears to help patients given the moderately emetic chemotherapeutic agents.

3. *Antihistamines* and *anticholinergics* apparently have little or no role to play in the management of cancer chemotherapy patients with nausea and vomiting.

4. *Cannabis, THC,* and *synthetic cannabinoids* like Nabilone and levonantradol have produced a much needed activity in the search for more effective antiemetics. Eleven controlled trials involving THC have been completed. In eight, THC was rated as better than either a placebo or Compazine.

Two investigations showed THC and Compazine to be equally efficacious, and in one study THC and Haldol were considered equally effective. Nabilone was believed to be better than Compazine in two clinical experiments. A number of controlled studies with levonantradol are under way. A recent supplement issue of the *Journal of Clinical Pharmacology*[4] summarizes the state of the art in cannabinoid therapeutic research.

Some investigators claim that the "high" is predictive of antiemetic action, but others do not find this to be so. Improvement may correlate with blood levels; the best results are obtained at 10 mg or more orally.

The average effective oral THC dose is 5 to 10 mg/M_2, or about 7.5 to 15 mg started two hours before the chemotherapy begins and repeated every four hours for 24 to 48 hours. Smoked material may be more reliable because of incomplete intestinal absorption.

The side effects of THC tend to be more upsetting than those of other antiemetics. Most patients notice drowsiness and dry mouth. A small number experience concentration difficulties, depersonalization, panicky states, or a brief psychotic reaction. A few investigators do not recommend THC as routine treatment because of the undesired effects. They suggest that it be used only if other medications fail.

It is presumed that the cannabinoids act centrally to raise the nausea/vomiting threshold of the emetic center. In one study[5] a combination of THC and Compazine performed better than either drug alone. While THC is not the final answer to chemotherapy-induced emesis, it does seem to help certain patients who do not respond to other antiemetics.

5. *Metoclopramide* (Reglan) is a procainamide (Pronestyl) derivative with the latter's effects on the heart rhythm. It has both peripheral and central antiemetic activity. The drug increases gastric tone and gastric emptying. In a recent study from the Sloan-Kettering Cancer Center,[6] when Reglan was given intravenously in much larger doses than those customarily used, it was an effective agent against the strongly emetic drug, cisplatin. The dosages were ten times the previously employed amounts, or between 150 to 200 mg every two hours. Reglan has significantly fewer episodes and shorter duration of vomiting, and it decreases the volume of emesis when compared with intramuscular Compazine or a placebo. Sedation was the most frequently encountered side effect. These studies have been confirmed in another series of over 100 patients.[7] Reglan must be considered a significant advance in antiemetic therapy because of its effect upon cisplatin nausea and vomiting. We can hope that it may also ameliorate the nausea and vomiting from other cancer chemotherapeutic agents.

6. Utilizing an entirely different rationale for control of the demoralizing effects of the retching and vomiting of anticancer drugs, parenteral *benzodiazepines* like Valium and Ativan have been used. These drugs only partially af-

fect the symptoms, but they do produce an amnesia for the noxious episode. This procedure has been used when no other way to control the distressing symptoms is available.

SUMMARY

The renewed attention paid to the distressing and debilitating symptoms of cancer chemotherapeutic agents is providing new drugs for their amelioration. THC is one of the helpful antiemetics, but its partial effectiveness and its adverse effects mean that it may have a definite, but restricted usefulness. It probably represents a transitional drug, with better cannabinoids eventually displacing it.

REFERENCES

1. Seigel, L.J. and Longo, D. The control of chemotherapy-induced emesis. Ann. Int. Med. 95:352, 1981.
2. Nesse, R.M. et al. Pretreatment nausea in cancer chemotherapy: A conditioned response? Psychosomatic Med. 42: 33, 1980.
3. Chang, J.C. Nausea and vomiting in cancer patients: An expression of psychological mechanisms? Psychosomatics. 22:707, 1981.
4. Therapeutic Progress in Cannabinoid Research. G.M. Milne et al., Eds. J. Clinical Pharmacol. 21 (Supplement) (Aug-Sep), 1981.
5. Garb, S. et al. Two-pronged study of THC prevention of vomiting from cancer chemotherapy. IRCS Med. Sci. 8: 203, 1980.
6. Gralla, R.J. Antiemetic activity of high dose metoclopramide: Randomized trials with placebo and prochlorperazine in patients with chemotherapy-induced nausea and vomiting. New Engl. J. Med. 305: 906, 1981.
7. Opfell, R. To be published.

III
THE ALCOHOL ISSUES

13. The Blood Alcohol Concentration

The blood alcohol concentration (BAC) or blood alcohol level (BAL) is a reliable and reproducible measurement of ethanol in the blood. Since alcohol diffuses uniformly to all tissues, it is also a reflection of brain cthanol levels. Breath alcohol determinations are more frequently used for practical purposes and converted by a factor of about 2,300 so that the apparatus automatically provides a BAC reading. Breath alcohol determinations should not be done within 15 minutes of having had a drink, otherwise false elevations will occur in some cases due to the retention of ingested alcohol in the oropharynx. Urine alcohol tests only generally reflect the BAC and are not worth performing for practical purposes.

BAC READINGS

Three different ways of reporting the BAC are used, and this may lead to occasional confusion. Examples of each are given below for the BAC that is legally assumed to be an intoxicating level.

G/100ml		mg/100ml		G/liter
or		or		or
		mg/dl		
		or		
%		mg/%		promille
0.1	=	100	=	1.0

In this chapter, percent will be used. It is converted to mg % by multiplying by 1,000. Promille is used in a number of foreign countries.

THE BAC AND DRIVING

The legal limit for intoxication throughout most of the United States is 0.1 percent. In some states this amount is presumptive evidence of intoxication, while in others it is *per se* evidence, meaning that a finding of 0.1 percent or above in itself proves intoxication. Supporting evidence is unnecessary for conviction. Most European countries have lowered their level to 0.08 percent or lower. The World Health Organization recommends a 0.05 percent limit. A number of investigators have found that driving skills start becoming impaired at 0.04 percent. By the time a BAC of 0.1 percent is reached the probability of auto accidents rises to seven or eight times the sober level.

The BAC determines the punishment for driving-while-intoxicated arrests in a country like Denmark. For BACs between 0.08 and 0.12 percent the fine is automatically a month's salary after taxes. From 0.121 to 0.15 percent it is a month's salary plus loss of one's driver's license for one year. When the BAC is found to be 0.151 or higher, the offender is imprisoned for 10 days, and loses his or her license for two years. Thus, the BAC is relied upon to mete out punishment. This may be one of the few instances where a biological test is used to determine the severity of a sentence.

THE BAC AND DRINKING

Although the BAC is quite reliable, the variance is ± 10 percent. Therefore, two tests are preferable to a single determination. The test is not a measure of the amount of ethanol consumed. The weight of the person is very important; also, the rapidity of drinking, the time elapsed since the last drink, the particular ability of the drinker to metabolize alcohol, the presence of food in the gastrointestinal tract, and other factors will determine the BAC. For example, a person weighing 100 pounds will have a BAC of about 0.22 after consuming five drinks within an hour. A 200-pound individual will have a BAC approximating 0.11 percent under the same circumstances.

A standard drink is defined as either 12 ounces of beer, 5 ounces of dry wine or 1½ ounces of 80 proof liquor. These quantities contain approximately the same amount of alcohol. Alcoholic beverages between 4 and 44 percent provide similar BACs. Below that percentage the alcohol absorption may be delayed by the large fluid volume. Above that percentage pylorospasm may delay absorption. The notion that whiskey produces drunkenness quicker than the more dilute beverages is probably due to the greater rapidity of its ingestion.

About 90 percent of the alcohol consumed is metabolized by liver-produced enzymes, particularly alcohol dehydrogenase. The rate of oxidation is fairly uniform for each person averaging 0.015 percent of the BAC per hour with a range of 0.012 to 0.018 percent. This is equivalent to the metabolism of 1 gram of pure alcohol for every 10 kg of body weight per hour.

The rate of destruction of alcohol is independent of the BAC except at levels above 0.3 percent when other enzymes like catalase and the microsomal endoplasmic oxidizing system of the liver come into play. The remaining 10 percent of the ingested alcohol is excreted unchanged by the lungs and kidneys with small amounts eliminated by the skin. It is difficult to accelerate the metabolism of alcohol, but physical exercise can increase it somewhat. The mechanism may be increased via breath and sweat excretion.

Although intestinal fermentation produces up to an ounce of ethanol a day the alcohol dehydrogenase system is efficient enough to immediately degrade it. Therefore a person who has taken no alcohol in beverage, medicinal, or food forms will have a BAC of 0 percent.

Since the rate of removal of alcohol from the blood is fairly constant, it is unnecessary to obtain a breath or blood sample immediately following an accident. If four hours have elapsed since an accident, and an estimate of the BAC at that time is desired, then a sample can be taken. To the reading that is obtained, 0.06 percent should be added (0.015 percent times 4 hours). The corrected figure will approximate the BAC at the time of the accident. Similarly if a person goes to sleep with a BAC of 0.15 and sleeps ten hours, he or she should awaken with a reading of 0 percent.

One possible error in such calculations will occur if considerable amounts of alcohol remained in the gastrointestinal tract at the time the BAC was tested. Metabolic breakdown of ethanol to acetaldehyde and acetate would continue. Meanwhile, additional amounts of alcohol would continue to be absorbed from the stomach and small intestine increasing the BAC, and that increase could not be predicted. To avoid such error, BAC samples should not be obtained until 20 minutes have elapsed since the last drink.

CLINICAL CORRELATES OF THE BAC

It has been claimed that some excessive drinkers have difficulties with alcohol because they are unable to self-monitor their BAC. The importance of this factor in drinking more than was planned is not known. Training patients who have occasional problems with overdrinking to discriminate their BACs have been attempted. They are given periodic feedback while drinking by telling them what their blood alcohol level is. Patients are given training in identifying the behavioral effects that typically accompany various BACs. They are required to discontinue their consumption at some specific upper level (typically 0.065 percent). Although some success with this method has been achieved, it is far from being a proven therapy, and should not be used with chronic alcoholics.

Recognizing the variability of the BAC according to the factors already mentioned, an attempt will be made to indicate some approximate clinical effects with increasing BACs. At 0.03 percent (one drink) most people will feel little or nothing. A few might note flushing and be somewhat more talkative than usual. At 0.05 percent (two drinks) some relaxation and lowering of inhibitions are observable in nontolerant drinkers. If four or five drinks are taken within an hour, a BAC of about 0.1 percent will be present. Most people will feel intoxicated at this level, others will deny intoxication but will do poorly on psychomotor testing, and a few, perhaps those with some partial tolerance, will show no evidence of ataxia, slurred speech, or mental confusion. At BACs of 0.15 to 0.3 percent (six to ten drinks), a staggering gait, passing out, blacking out, or irrational behavior can occur. A BAC of 0.35 has been considered to be the LD_{50} for alcohol (a lethal dose for 50 percent of the population), but this figure has been disputed by others as too low. They suggest a level of 0.4 percent at which point the person is comatose. On the other hand alcoholics have been known who survived a reading of 0.5 percent or more. Such BACs can be obtained by drinking a quart of whiskey in an hour. Drinkers who have achieved tolerance to alcohol manifest less effect than nontolerant ones at every BAC.

These approximations are given for determinations done during the ascending limb of the BAC curve. During this period the mental effects are more pronounced and the mood tends to be more euphoric. On the other hand, as the BAC declines, at equivalent blood levels the mental effects are less pronounced and less pleasant feeling tones are experienced. The explanation of this finding, and it has been consistently reported, is not evident.

Lateral nystagmus correlates quite well with the BAC. At high BAC levels nystagmus is observed on direct gaze. At lower BACs nystagmus can be elicited by fixing on an object on the lateral periphery. With precise measurement of this phenomenon, the degree of lateral fixing that produces nystagmus can provide an estimate of the BAC. Other CNS depressants can also cause lateral nystagmus.

The National Council on Alcoholism criteria for the diagnosis of alcoholism include the following. A BAC of 0.15 percent or more in the absence of gross intoxication is definitely indicative of marked tolerance and therefore of alcoholism. A BAC of 0.1 percent encountered during a routine examination is a minor sign suggestive of alcoholism. A BAC of 0.3 percent at any time is also one of the minor signs that contributes to a diagnosis of alcoholism.

USES OF THE BAC

Traffic Safety

The BAC is a primary instrument in a number of aspects of motor vehicle safety control. Unsafe driving such as weaving or speeding might call for a BAC test. Accidents, especially serious ones, often require blood alcohol determinations. Routine roadside surveys take a blood or breath sample to determine the alcohol usage of a random sample of auto operators.

The BAC test is an important tool in dealing with those drivers while under the influence. It provides objective evidence that supports or refutes the arresting officer's evaluation of the car operator. A BAC, and particularly two determinations, are given considerable weight in court and during sentencing. The mere ability to do the test has doubtless served as a deterrent to some intoxicated persons who consider driving.

Self-administered breath alcohol analyzers are available so vehicle operators can check their own alcohol levels before driving. A few bars also have such portable analyzers available. Some research has been done to build breath testing or cognitive tasks into the ignition system of a car that could prevent the car from starting if the test is failed.

Court Procedures

The BAC is helpful in determining the degree of impairment so that an opinion can be formed about the specific intent to commit a criminal act. Although a 0.1 percent BAC is legal evidence of intoxication, such a level would be insufficient to make a defendant incapable of premeditating, reflecting upon, harboring malice, or of being able to form the intent to commit the crime of which he or she is accused. Furthermore, a plea of diminished capacity is not a valid defense when the defendant knew that drinking alcohol could produce a disturbed mental state. If involuntary intoxication can be proven, for example, drinking under duress, then the Durham Rule would hold. This rule states that the accused is not criminally responsible if the unlawful act was the product of mental disease or a mental defect.

Research

A good deal of the biobehavioral research on alcohol uses repeated BACs to correlate with the physiologic or psychologic changes that take place. The breath and blood tests are accurate enough to be used for research purposes.

Diagnosis and Treatment

Emergency rooms often use the BAC in instances of injuries. One study has reported that in fights one or both contestants have measurable blood levels 55 percent of the time. Some physicians check breath or blood levels on routine visits. The breath procedure is quickly done and inexpensive. During the treatment of an alcoholic patient such testing is performed to provide an objective measure of recent compliance. Other physicians will not do the test because of a concern that it interferes with the patient-physician relationship. If the arrangement is set up as a part of the treatment contract at the outset, it is usually acceptable to the patient. Methadone maintenance clinics may do the BAC routinely, at random, or when specifically indicated.

A person first seen in coma and with the odor of alcohol on his or her breath, should have a BAC performed to rule alcohol in or out as the cause of the coma. Many other causes of coma may be masked and remain undiagnosed if the obvious cause, alcohol, is accepted. The odor of acetone in a patient in diabetic coma resembles that of alcohol on a person's breath.

Personnel Management

Some firms include BAC testing in their drug screening program of preemployment physicals. It is sometimes done in the medical departments of corporations in order to clarify unusual on-the-job accidents or bizarre behavior. If suspension or dismissal action is contemplated, it is desirable to have objective evidence like a BAC test of intoxication during working hours.

14. Hangover

Hangovers, a source of misery for those who have them and of amusement for those nearby, rarely require medical attention. Nevertheless, they provide an interesting component of the varieties of alcohol experiences.

The causes and consequences of the hungover state following immoderate alcohol consumption have not been completely clarified. Although it is a frequent event, the hangover has, until recently, not been as thoroughly studied as some of the other alcohol-related conditions. It is a self-limited disorder and despite the appreciable distress involved, it is ordinarily treated with folk remedies. Much of the current research on this postintoxication state comes from Finland where it is recognized as a considerable cause of absenteeism and decreased productivity.

SYMPTOMS AND SIGNS

This unpleasant interlude, following acute alcohol intoxication by 8 to 12 hours, has a long list of manifestations. Perhaps the most frequently encountered is a splitting headache, made worse by movement, bright lights, and loud sounds. Upper gastrointestinal symptoms of heartburn, loss of appetite, nausea, and vomiting are frequent. Dry mouth and a severe thirst are annoying and common. Nystagmus can be observed, and interestingly enough, it is opposite in direction to the to-and-fro movements of the eye seen during the acute intoxicated state.

In addition to the headache, other central nervous system and autonomic system side effects include dizziness, sweating, tremulousness, pallor, palpitations, and sometimes insomnia. During this period either anxiety or depression or both may be noted. Generalized symptoms of malaise and tiredness are frequent complaints.

CAUSES AND CONSEQUENCES

This array of symptoms and signs can hardly result from some single cause. The present idea about the etiology of the hangover is that a number of contributing factors combines to produce the picture with certain factors being dominant in specific instances. Needless to say, what is presented here should be seen as an interim explanation of the postalcoholic syndrome.

The Stress Response

Acute alcoholic intoxication is a physiologically stressful condition, made worse by associated factors such as lack of sleep, heavy smoking, and various feelings evoked by one's uninhibited behavior. A nonspecific adrenergic response can be measured that precipitates a release of ACTH and cortisol and, perhaps, increased hypothalamic dopaminergic activity leading to a secondary inhibition of dopamine release. Moreover, elevated free fatty acid and triglyceride levels correlate quite well with the severity of hangover. These are changes that are expected following a stress reaction. Plasma testosterone levels are also known to be depressed during stress, and they are found to be lower during the postintoxication state.

Whether any of these endocrine shifts produces actual symptoms of hangover is not known but they may contribute to their severity.

Hypoglycemia

Many of the manifestations of the hangover are reminiscent of hypoglycemia. Ethanol is known to lower blood glucose concentrations in the fasting state. In addition, not eating and vomiting add to the reduction of available carbohydrates. The blood glucose levels are at their lowest at the height of the hangover, but no differences in glucose concentrations are detectable between the mild and the severe hangovers. Therefore, in itself, hypoglycemia may worsen the postintoxication syndrome, but is only infrequently a primary cause of the state.

Acidosis

It is well established that ethanol produces a metabolic, and occasionally a respiratory acidosis. The pH of the blood falls significantly during the hangover phase, at the same time blood lactate and total ketone bodies are rising. The accumulation of organic acids and ketones resulting from the degradation of ethanol in the liver accounts for the ketoacidosis. The degree of acidosis correlates fairly well with the hangover's intensity and may be at least partially involved in its genesis. Fructose, a sugar currently in favor for the treatment of hangover, will reduce ketone body concentrations and also return blood pH and glucose levels to normal. But in controlled studies fructose had no measurable effect on the intensity of either the acute intoxicated or the postintoxicated state.

Acetaldehyde

Some of the effects of the postintoxication syndrome resemble the alcohol-Antabuse reaction which is manifested by high acetaldehyde levels. Therefore it is natural to look at acetaldehyde as a possible cause. It was found that the blood acetaldehyde curve was similar to the ethanol curve so that all the acetaldehyde had been eliminated before the hangover began. Thus, acetaldehyde hardly can be a major etiologic factor in hangover induction.

Dehydration and Hyperhydration

A good candidate for a supporting role in the pathogenesis of hangovers is water balance alterations. It has been amply confirmed that alcohol intake decreases, then increases the secretion of the antidiuretic hormone vasopressin from the posterior pituitary gland. This leads to a retention and later a diuresis of urine. Although much fluid may be ingested during a drinking bout, more will be voided. The increased urinary excretion can lead to dehydration. In addition, water loss during sweating, vomiting, and diarrhea will add to the fluid depletion, symptomatically manifested as dry mouth and thirst. On the other hand, as blood alcohol levels drop, antidiuretic hormone is stimulated, and hyperhydration can develop during the hangover.

Congeners

The congeners (fusel oil) are organic alcohols and salts formed when alcoholic beverages are manufactured. They include methanol, propanol, butyl and amyl alcohol, ethyl acetate, and ethyl formate. Vodkas, which are essentially diluted alcohol, contain the least, and bourbons and brandies contain the most fusel oil. Congeners provide the flavor and aroma of the beverage.

Congeners have been suspected of hangover production for some time. But they are present in only small amounts and can hardly play an important role. Furthermore, pure ethanol has been amply shown to induce the hungover state. At most, fusel oil can only contribute to the condition by competing with ethyl alcohol for its metabolizing enzyme, alcohol dehydrogenase.

Local Toxic Effects of Alcohol

The gastrointestinal upset, a prominent hangover feature, may be directly produced by alcohol, especially in its more concentrated forms. Alcohol stimulates the secretion of hydrochloric acid and is known to produce inflammatory and erosive changes of the stomach lining. The nausea and vomiting may be a result of an acute gastritis that follows one or more heavy encounters with ethanol.

Alcohol

It appears that a necessary, but not a sufficient condition for causing a hangover, is a large enough quantity of alcohol. Some heavy drinkers, though, claim never to have had one, but other consumers complain of distressing "morning after" disturbances following rather moderate imbibing. Some of this variance may be related to psychological factors. It has been found that those drinkers who had negative attitudes toward drinking had more severe hangover symptoms than those with positive attitudes toward their drinking.

Although it is generally believed that the amount consumed relates to the appearance and severity of the hangover, no study could be found to prove the point. As indicated, the hangover probably has a multifactorial etiology, with alcohol being the major element involved.

The central role of alcohol in the development of hangovers is underlined by a number of alcohologists who believe that the postintoxication syndrome is a manifestation of early withdrawal. Even after a single drinking bout a certain degree of tolerance develops. As evidence for this point of view, they cite the different responses to the blood alcohol concentration (BAC) on the ascending part of the curve to the lessened response on the descending limb of the BAC. The symptoms are viewed as rebound withdrawal effects. The fact that resuming drinking will reverse the symptomatology is cited as additional evidence for the concept.

TREATMENT

The "hair of the dog that bit you" treatment of the hangover is a traditional one. This use of a small amount of alcohol to correct the metabolic rebound is justifiable if it does not lead to another round of overdrinking. It is also rational if we accept the early withdrawal concept of the hangover.

To correct the acidosis, water balance disturbance, and low blood sugar, fluids such as orange juice would seem indicated. Rest and time will correct the other changes induced by the overindulgence. There is no objection to mild analgesics for the hangover headache. Sedatives and tranquilizers are not indicated.

SUMMARY

It would be interesting to know whether anyone has ever stopped drinking because of one or more severe hangovers. If so, then hangovers may have a protective quality for some people. On the other hand their punishing psychophysical effects may serve to reinforce a dysfunctional drinking pattern since relief is obtained by returning to alcohol.

The causes of the hangover are multiple but alcohol is a necessary element. Other factors intervene to determine the nature and extent of the symptoms. The notion that we are dealing with an early alcohol withdrawal syndrome is worth exploring further. Not all aspects of the postalcoholic states can be dealt with at this time.

BIBLIOGRAPHY

- Anylian G.H., Dorn, J. and Swerdlow, J. The manifestations and assessment of ethanol-induced hangover. South African Med. J. 54:193, 1978.
- Linkola, J., Fykrquist, F. and Ylikahri, R.H. Renin, aldosterone and cortisol during ethanol intoxication and hangover. Acta Physiol. Scand. 106:75, 1979.
- Ylikahri, R.H. and Huttunen, M.U. Metabolic and endocrine pathology during hangover. In: *Alcohol Intoxication and Withdrawal IIIb*, Ed.: M.M. Gross, Plenum, N.Y., 1977.

15. Alcoholic Hypoglycemia

Hypoglycemia is both an overdiagnosed and underdiagnosed condition. Since many of the symptoms resemble an anxiety attack or other sort of "nervous" reaction, the two conditions may be misidentified with each other.

It is not surprising that hypoglycemia presents with symptoms of anxiety. As blood sugar levels drop, adrenalin secretion is stimulated, producing a mobilization of glycogen stores with an increased availability of glucose. Adrenalin also causes tenseness, sweating, faintness, hunger, tachycardia, and tremulousness.

Other evidences of hypoglycemia are due to the cortical depression from a very low blood sugar, and they include confusion, visual disturbances, ataxia, headache, muscle weakness, convulsions, and coma. A fasting blood sugar level of 40 mg percent or under, and a rapid response to intravenous or oral sugar is confirmatory diagnostic evidence. Sometimes a three- or five-hour glucose tolerance test is needed to provoke low blood sugar levels when the patient is seen between attacks. In severe cases the blood sugar level has dropped to as low as 5 mg percent.

ALCOHOL AND HYPOGLYCEMIA

The causes of hypoglycemia are many (see Table 15–1), but we will focus here on the relationships between alcohol consumption and hypoglycemic episodes. One report estimates that 70 percent of all reactive hypoglycemias are induced by alcohol. Some of the symptoms mentioned are reminiscent of certain alcoholic states. For example, the acute intoxicated condition, the delirium tremens, and chronic inebriation all may resemble some of the manifestations of hypoglycemia. Stupor and coma in a person who has been drinking must be quickly differentiated, because untreated, extremely low blood sugar levels are incompatible with survival. Some people whose autonomic or neurologic symptoms and signs exceed the amount of ethyl alcohol consumed, should be suspected of having hypoglycemia.

Even the sober, convalescent alcoholic may have a low blood sugar level. During sobriety he or she may remain with an unstable glucose-regulating

Table 15-1
The Differential Diagnosis of Hypoglycemia

I. **Exogenous (Reactive) Causes**
   A. High intake or rapid absorption of carbohydrate
      1. Insulin overshoot hypoglycemia
      2. Postgastrectomy syndrome (dumping syndrome)
   B. Inhibition of glycogenolysis by specific nutrients
      1. Fructose intolerance
      2. Galactosemia
      3. Leucine sensitivity (maple syrup urine disease)
   C. Drugs
      1. Excess glucose utilization
         a. Excessive insulin administration
         b. Insulin effect intensified by propanolol, oxytetracyline, EDTA, manganese, etc.
         c. Excessive sulfonurea administration
         d. Sulfonurea effect intensified by sulfa drugs, dicumarol, phenylbutazone, and alcohol
         e. Excess phenformin administration
      2. Deficient glucose production
         a. Alcohol
         b. Salicylates
         c. Aminobenzoic acid
         d. Chlorpromazine
         e. Haloperidol
         f. Propoxyphene

II. **Endogenous (Spontaneous) Causes**
   A. Excess glucose utilization
      1. Insulinoma (tumor of pancreatic beta cells)
      2. Deficiency of anti-insulin hormones: glucagon, cortisol, epinephrine, growth and thyroid hormones
      3. Neonatal hypoglycemia of infants born of diabetic mothers.
   B. Excessive glucose utilization or excretion
      1. Exercise
      2. Fever
      3. Pregnancy
      4. Renal glycosuria
      5. Certain tumors may utilize large amounts of glucose
   C. Deficient glucose production
      1. Liver disease
      2. Glycogen mobilization disorder (glycogen storage disease)
      3. Glucose-6-phosphate deficiency (poor glucose release)
      4. Fructose-1-6-diphosphotase deficiency

mechanism that produces weakness, headache, a rapid pulse, sweating, hunger feelings, and anxiety. This usually occurs many hours after a carbohydrate-rich meal and is associated with a craving for coffee, sweets, and soft drinks. Unless the distressing symptoms are brought under control, they may provoke a relapse.

ALCOHOLIC HYPOGLYCEMIA: MECHANISMS

Alcohol ingestion does many things to carbohydrate metabolism, some of which culminate in reduced levels of circulating glucose. In healthy drinkers small amounts of alcohol produce a mild initial hyperglycemia possibly due to the carbohydrate-sparing effect of the drug, or because of alcohol's release of catecholamines that provokes glycogenolysis (liver glycogen breakdown to glucose). The elevated circulating glucose stimulates the beta cells of the pancreas to secrete insulin. If the person is sensitive to the glucose-lowering effects of insulin, mild hypoglycemia could result.

What is more common is that malnourished or fasting drinkers whose glycogen stores are greatly depleted will experience hypoglycemia even in the absence of liver disease. The hypoglycemic episode typically occurs after four or more hours of drinking. Since glucose and glycogen are readily manufactured from proteins and fats, it is apparent that gluconeogenesis (the synthesis of glucose from amino acids in protein and glycerol in fat) is also adversely affected by alcohol. This occurs because in the metabolism of alcohol and acetaldehyde, hydrogen ions are produced. The latter are immediately bound to NAD (nicotinamide adenine dinucleotide) to form $NADH_2$. The $NADH_2$ drives the chemical reactions toward lactate and away from the precursors of carbohydrate, like pyruvate.

Severe alcoholic liver damage can compound the distortions of carbohydrate metabolism. Glycogen is poorly stored in necrotic hepatocytes. But hypoglycemia only occurs in end-stage cirrhosis. More commonly, hyperglycemia and frank diabetes develop as a result of alcoholic hepatitis and cirrhosis. This is attributed to a resistance to circulating insulin and is detectable in glucose and insulin tolerance tests. Insulin resistance may be secondary to increased amounts of circulating growth hormone, an insulin antagonist known to be elevated in cirrhotics. Chronic alcoholic pancreatitis also will cause diabetes, and this complication is evidently induced by diminished insulin production by the beta cells.

Pathologic drinking practices eventually will affect the intestine's ability to absorb carbohydrates and other nutrients by damage to the mucosa and deficiencies of the digestive enzymes of the pancreas. This end effect is similar to starvation or malnutrition, a contributory factor to hypoglycemia. Gastritis, associated with anorexia and vomiting, and the steatorrhea of the malabsorption syndrome also reduce carbohydrate absorption.

PREVENTION AND TREATMENT

Not only may severe hypoglycemia end fatally, but recurrent attacks can result in brain injury since glucose is the nerve cell's only nutritional substrate. Therefore the termination and correction of such attacks are important. For those who sustain hypoglycemic episodes in connection with their alcohol use, abstention or a marked reduction in the amount consumed is strongly recommended. This step alone may eliminate the problem. If it does not, four to six small meals daily should be eaten. They should be low in carbohydrates and high in fat and protein in order not to stimulate insulin release. Caffeine is interdicted by some physicians and for the same reason. For the acute attack intravenous glucose will be necessary if the patient cannot swallow. Fruit juices with added sugar are generally given by mouth to those whose symptoms are not severe.

Hypoglycemia is another reason why drinkers should not drive. The confusion, faintness, dizziness, and impaired psychomotor skills can lead to driving mishaps. If an incident that can be identified as hypoglycemia occurs while driving, the individual should pull over and stop as soon as it is safely possible, obtain some sugar-containing food, and consume it. Relief ought to be noticeable within 10 minutes. People who have experienced a number of attacks usually keep a few chocolate bars in the glove compartment.

SUMMARY

When the symptoms of people who have been drinking exceed what would be expected from their blood alcohol concentration, hypoglycemia is one of the possibilities that should be considered. This is especially true in instances of coma associated with the consumption of alcoholic beverages. Those who have experienced hypoglycemic attacks while sober are well advised to avoid overindulgence in ethanol. Drinkers who sustain such episodes ought to be cautioned to abstain or reduce their intake markedly.

Physicians must always consider the possibility of hypoglycemic stupor or coma in an unconscious person smelling of alcohol. A trial injection of glucose might be indicated as a diagnostic aid. People with insulin-producing tumors and with alcohol on their breath have been labelled drunks because of the bizarre behavior evoked by their very low blood sugar.

High alcohol intake can produce the following carbohydrate shifts and cause hypoglycemia:

1. Decreased intake or loss of nutrients.

2. Impaired absorption of carbohydrates and vitamins needed for carbohydrate metabolism.

3. Diversion of pyruvate to lactate preventing gluconeogenesis.

4. Reduction of liver glycogen stores.

5. Indirect stimulation of insulin secretion.

BIBLIOGRAPHY

- Baruh, S. et al. Fasting hypoglycemia. Med. Clin. N. Amer. 57: 1441-1462, 1973.
- Cohen, S. A review of hypoglycemia and alcoholism with or without liver disease. Ann. N.Y. Acad. Sci. 273:338-342, 1976.
- Jaffe, B. et al. Hormonal response in ethanol-induced hypoglycemia. J. Studies Alcohol. 36:550-554, 1975.
- Kissin, B. and Begleiter, H. *The Biology of Alcoholism*, Vol. 1: Biochemistry. Plenum, N.Y., 1971.
- Leggett, J. and Favazza, A. R. Hypoglycemia: An overview. J. Clin. Psychiat. 39:51-57, 1978.
- Nikkola, E. A. and Taskinen, M. R. Ethanol-induced alterations of glucose tolerance, postglucose hypoglycemia and insulin secretion. Diabetes. 24:933-943, 1975.
- Ragnar, H. et al. Does a disturbed insulin release promote hypoglycemia in alcoholics? Acta. Med. Scand. 204:57-60, 1978.
- Searle, G. et al. Evaluation of ethanol hypoglycemia in man. Metabolism. 23:1023-1035, 1974.

16. The Oriental Syndrome

A large number of Orientals have a sensitivity to alcoholic beverages that is manifested by a marked facial flush shortly after consuming even small amounts. Some American Indians, East Europeans, and members of other cultures may show a similar hypersensitivity to ethanol. As little as one drink might bring on the temporary reddening of the face, neck, and, sometimes, the upper chest.

Along with the dilation of the skin capillaries, some highly sensitive individuals, or those who imbibe large amounts of alcohol, manifest additional autonomic symptoms. Hypotension, tachycardia, and bronchoconstriction can occur, and the person may feel exceedingly uncomfortable.

The flush may vary from a mild reddening of the skin around the mouth to severe flushing over the upper third of the body. Symptoms like dizziness, sleepiness, pounding in the head, and nausea are apt to accompany the cutaneous manifestations. Orientals who do not flush may experience certain of these generalized symptoms more often than non-Orientals after equivalent amounts of alcohol.

The flush syndrome has been cited as an important reason why the incidence of alcoholism in Orientals may be lower than that of other races. Of course, other factors must play important roles, but the inability to drink large amounts comfortably may reinforce sociocultural influences.

Those who exhibit the flush syndrome tend to be either abstainers or modest drinkers, due to their physiologic intolerance. Large quantities, however, are taken by some sensitive individuals who run the risk of asthmatic attacks or cardiovascular collapse. The problems that a number of American Indians have with excessive drinking points out that physiologic discomfort is not necessarily a bar to heavy alcohol consumption. Actually, no investigation has been done to determine whether Indian flushers are less likely to consume large amounts of alcoholic beverages than nonflushing Indians.

ETIOLOGY

The precise cause of this aberration of alcohol metabolism is unknown, but a genetic component is undoubtedly involved. It has been assumed that a reduction or an absence of the enzyme aldehyde dehydrogenase produces a retention of acetaldehyde. Acetaldehyde is the first metabolic product of alcohol and is much more toxic than ethanol itself. The accumulation of acetaldehyde in the body could account for the unpleasant symptoms of the Oriental flush syndrome. Although flushers have higher blood acetaldehyde levels than nonflushers, the elevation is not marked, and acetaldehyde may not be a complete explanation of the phenomenon. The release of biogenic amines like norepinephrine, histamine, and serotonin also occurs, but these might be the result of the stressful flush reaction rather than a cause of it.

ANTABUSE AND RELATED DRUGS

It is well established that disulfiram (Antabuse) and other alcohol-sensitizing drugs increase blood acetaldehyde levels due to an inhibition of aldehyde dehydrogenase. Other compounds that act in a like manner, although not as efficiently, are citrated calcium carbamide (Temposil) and sulfonylurea compounds like Orinase.

The symptoms of the alcohol-Antabuse reaction are rather similar to the flush syndrome but may be more intense depending on the alcohol and the Antabuse dosages. The Physicians Desk Reference[1] describes the reaction as follows: "flushing, throbbing in head and neck, throbbing headache, respiratory difficulty, nausea, copious vomiting, sweating, thirst, chest pain, palpitation, dyspnea, hyperventilation, tachycardia, hypotension, marked uneasiness, weakness, vertigo, blurred vision and confusion. In severe reactions there may be respiratory depression, cardiovascular collapse, myocardial infarction, acute congestive heart failure, unconsciousness, convulsions and death."

It has been speculated that alcohol-sensitive persons have a built-in alcohol-Antabuse situation that should protect them from overdrinking, but it does not always do so. Patients on Antabuse have deliberately challenged its deterrent effect on occasion by drinking alcohol. Some people will drink wood alcohol, rubbing alcohol, fusel oil, and other toxic concoctions indicating that pleasurable effects are not a requirement for drinking intoxicants, nor are noxious effects a bar. Apparently the rewards of intoxication outweigh the aversive effects for these people.

ACETALDEHYDE

Acetaldehyde has been accused of much of the toxic impact of heavy alcohol consumption. For example, the hangovers, alcoholic cardiomyopathy, alcoholic liver injury, and impaired protein synthesis in alcoholics have been related to acetaldehyde. These assumptions are based upon the fact that acetaldehyde is 10 to 20 times more toxic than ethyl alcohol. No evidence for a fetal acetaldehyde syndrome has been claimed, perhaps because the placenta is very efficient in oxidizing acetaldehyde to acetate.

The problem is that while acetaldehyde can induce most of the symptoms of the flush syndrome, it does so at blood levels higher than that found in people who are flushing. The suggestion has been made that the high initial spike of acetaldehyde production a few minutes after alcohol intake might produce flushing. This may take place due to a surge of ethanol transformation to acetaldehyde because of a highly active alcohol dehydrogenase that is commonly found in the Japanese population.[2]

Thus the flush response could be caused by a relative decrease in the activity of acetaldehyde dehydrogenase or a relative increase in the activity of alcohol dehydrogenase. A third possibility is that the end organ (the skin capillaries over the blush area) is highly sensitive to ordinary amounts of acetaldehyde.

Animal studies have shown that compounds that produce an accumulation of acetaldehyde in the organism will cause the animals to restrict their drinking in a free-choice situation. Furthermore, the differences in alcohol consumption between genetically different strains of mice are directly related to differences in the way that they metabolize alcohol and acetaldehyde.

HISTAMINE

Another chemical candidate for the genesis of the flush response is histamine. As will be indicated, alcohol-sensitive people can develop hives over the blush area. This may be modulated by a release of histamine that dilates the skin capillaries and increases their permeability. Histamine is known to produce headache (histamine headache), a pulsating fullness in the head, bronchoconstriction, tachycardia, and hypotension (anaphylactic shock). Despite the overlap of symptoms, there is a little proof that histamine release is the primary cause of the flush syndrome.

RESEARCH STUDIES

In one study[3] 55 Chinese and Japanese men swallowed about one ounce of ethanol (0.4 ml/kg) in a 19 percent solution. Thirty-three (60 percent) developed a cutaneous flush, some of them had hives. Of 11 Caucasians only one (9 percent) flushed, and it was noted as mild. The only highly significant biochemical difference between flushers and nonflushers was a lower serum hydrocortisone level in the former group.

The decreased hydrocortisone response among Orientals as compared with Occidentals was also significant, but this was seen as a secondary effect of the exposure to the flush provocation test. In this study the mean acetaldehyde blood level of all Orientals was higher than among the Occidentals (p <.05) 30 minutes after drinking alcohol. Plasma histamine levels were not detectable in either group, nor were skin tests for alcohol positive.

Ewing and his colleagues[4] reported that in 24 persons of Oriental parentage, 17 (70 percent) showed a facial flush following use of alcohol. In 24 Caucasian men and women three (12.5 percent) demonstrated a flush. Capillary blood flow to the skin increased in the flushers, some had drops of systolic blood pressure in excess of 10 mm Hg. A mild tachycardia was recorded. Symptoms such as pounding in the head, muscle weakness, and dizziness were mentioned. Many more Orientals reported family members who flushed than did Occidental subjects.

A study[5] that compared 656 Chinese, 645 Japanese, 444 Hapa Haoles (one Oriental and one Caucasian parent), and 674 Caucasians, all living in Hawaii, revealed a much larger proportion of Orientals who flushed after drinking. Hapa Haoles had approximately the same percentage of flushers as the Oriental group. A greater percentage of Orientals reported no use of alcohol, possibly because of the unpleasant reaction. Causasians drank much more, and Hapa Haoles were intermediate in their alcohol consumption.

American Indians also have a higher rate of flushing than people of European extraction according to Wolff.[6] This is quite reasonable in view of the Mongoloid derivation of the Amerindians and their prehistoric migration across the Bering Strait. Fifty Caucasoids, 30 Cree Indians, 20 half-Mongoloid-half-Caucasoids, 15 Americans of Chinese or Japanese origin, and a small number of $\frac{1}{4}$-Mongoloid and $\frac{3}{4}$-Caucasoids were tested with an alcohol challenge. Visible flushing appeared in 4 percent of the Caucasoids, 50 percent of the Indians, 80 percent of the pure Orientals, 90 percent of those with half-Mongoloid ancestry, and 75 percent of those of $\frac{1}{4}$-Mongoloid extraction. The flush appeared within a few minutes. No male-female differences were noted. It would seem that the genotype for flushing is a dominant, since $\frac{1}{4}$ and $\frac{1}{2}$-Mongoloids inherit the trait in a high proportion of instances. In order to eliminate a placebo response, some of those who flushed after oral alcoholic beverages were administered either an intravenous alcohol solution or saline. Flushing occurred only when the alcohol was injected.

Wolff also reported that when tiny amounts of port wine in a glucose solution were given to Oriental infants, 74 percent flushed. The same preparation caused flushing in only 5 percent of Occidental infants. He concluded that dietary or cultural factors did not account for the differences between Orientals and Occidentals.

Twenty-six Japanese were given 200 ml of sake (a wine made of fermented rice) during a 10-minute period.

Of these, 11 flushed and 15 did not. Those who flushed had a significantly higher acetaldehyde blood level than those who did not. This is contrary to a number of studies that reported no relationship between acetaldehyde level and flushing.

SUMMARY

Many people of Mongolian ancestry metabolize alcohol in a manner that produces flushing and sometimes physiologic symptoms. This does not seem to protect many of them from excessive drinking since the rates of alcoholism have increased, particularly in Japan.[7] Furthermore, the American Indians who share the flush response because of their Mongolian lineage also have substantial problems with alcohol consumption.

REFERENCES

1. *Physicians Desk Reference*, 38th Edition, Medical Economics Co., Oradell, NJ, 1984, p. 629.
2. Lundros, K.O. Acetaldehyde—Its metabolism and role in the actions of alcohol. In: *Research Advances in Alcohol and Drug Problems,* Vol. II. Ed.: Israel, Y., et al., Plenum, New York, 1978, pp. 111-176.
3. Seto, H., et al. Biochemical correlates of ethanol-induced flushing in Orientals. J. Stud. Alcohol. 39:1-11, 1978.
4. Ewing, J.A., et al. Alcohol sensitivity and ethnic background. Am. J. Psychiatry. 131:206-210, 1974.
5. Wilson, J.R., et al. Ethnic variation in use and effects of alcohol. Drug & Alcohol Dependence. 3:147-151, 1978.
6. Wolff, P.H. Vasomotor sensitivity to alcohol in diverse mongoloid populations. Am. J. Human Genetics. 25:193-199, 1973.
7. Mendelson, J.H. and Mello, N.K. Biologic Concomitant of Alcoholism. New England Journal of Medicine. 301:912, 1979.

17. Blackouts: "You Mean I Did That Last Night?"

The amnesia (blackout) that follows the drinking of large amounts of alcoholic beverages is an important medical and legal matter. Blackouts can be defined as the inability to remember a part or all of a drinking episode even though consciousness was neither significantly clouded nor lost.

An alcoholic grayout is an intoxicated state after which recent prior events can be recalled, but with difficulty. Passing out consists of becoming stuporous or comatose in connection with drinking and, therefore, having no memory for anything that may have happened.

PHENOMENOLOGY

Blackouts can occur in both nonalcoholics and alcoholics who have drunk a good deal. In fact, Jellinek and others have considered these acute anterograde amnesias to be a prodromal sign of chronic alcoholism. Jellinek's triad of early alcohol addiction consisted of blackouts, benders, and loss of control, with blackouts usually appearing before the other two manifestations.

Predisposing factors include gulping drinks and not eating, suggesting that it is a rapid rise in the blood alcohol concentration that induces the amnesia. However, a blackout may become evident only after the first few days of binge drinking. Lack of sleep plays a role in its induction. Those who have sustained a blackout are likely to have subsequent ones. Some people report that they experience them on every episode of heavy drinking. Other heavy drinkers never seem to have blackouts. The highest incidence of blackouts occurs in those heavy drinkers who have considerable craving, who have a tolerance to alcohol, and who are solitary, gulping drinkers. In Tarter and Sugerman's series loss of control, head trauma, and whiskey drinking were found to be positive factors. A family history of blackouts was not correlated with the condition. This group of alcoholic patients was separated into cravers and noncravers of alcohol. Blackouts were reported by the cravers as follows: never 15.5 percent, sometimes 48.3 percent, often 22.4 percent, and almost every time 13.8 percent. The noncravers had fewer blackouts with 35.3 percent responding never, 58.8 percent saying sometimes, and the remaining 5.9 percent reporting almost every time.

The amnesic intervals can last for days or for shorter blocks of time. They are not restricted to certain significant events; instead they consist of a complete memory loss for everything that happened. Neither the persons involved nor those around them are ordinarily aware of the memory defect. They may go through the motions of functioning adequately and may not even seem very intoxicated to others.

Meanwhile, the blood alcohol level will be between 150 and 300 mg/dl. Generally, the drinkers will awaken after sleeping it off and be unable to remember what happened the evening before. If the events are related to them in detail, they will still not be able to recall them. If nothing of note happened, and witnesses do not try to remind them, they may not be aware that a blackout occurred.

During the state, a person functions more or less adequately, conversing, driving, and performing other well-learned acts. Someone may start drinking in Los Angeles and awaken in a hotel room in St. Louis a few days later quite unable to remember how he or she arrived there or anything that happened during the period.

Such profound memorial deficits can be accounted for by an inability to transfer short-term memories to long-term storage sites. The person is able to continue to perform because immediate memory—up to a minute—is retained, and the retrieval of information from the long-term memory banks is only partially disturbed. It is the transfer process of short-term data (what happened more than a minute ago) to the permanent memory stores that is knocked out. Thus a memory gap exists, and it cannot be filled in by cueing the person, or by attempting to retrieve the missing information under hypnosis or sodium pentothal.

It is entirely possible that alcoholic blackouts are much more common than we assume. A brief memory gap lasting minutes may not come to awareness, and even long ones may be ignored.

A lesser condition that could be called cocktail party transient and partial amnesia becomes observable when the drinker later tries to remember the contents of what seemed to be a significant conversation at the time. Memory losses occur in nonalcoholic drinkers after considerably lower doses than those associated with the blackout. A decreased ability to recall may take place at blood alcohol levels of 40 mg/dl, and it progresses in a linear fashion as the level rises.

CAUSATION

We can say what blackouts are not, but do not know what causes them. They are not the psychological repression of traumatic, "forgotten" incidents. They are usually not instances of state-dependent learning, since recall for the amnesic period will not take place during subsequent intoxications. They are not produced by structural alterations in the brain, since they are readily reversible, and tests of short-term memory function under sober conditions are within normal limits. Hypoglycemia has been ruled out as a causative factor.

Alcohol is one of the few substances known that induces substantial memory gaps in the presence of a consciousness that is relatively unimpaired. Puromycin, an antineoplastic and antitrypanosomal antibiotic, has also been shown to impair the storage of data into the memory banks, apparently by interfering with protein metabolism, specifically RNA. The metabolism of the processing of new information and of the storage process is probably disturbed when sufficient concentrations of alcohol are in contact with brain cells involved in the transfer process.

An interesting speculation deals with the relationship of blackouts, presumably a toxic process, to the amnestic-confabulatory syndrome of Wernicke-Korsakoff. The latter is an organic condition, usually caused in this country by chronic, heavy drinking and more precisely by the thiamine deficiency that accompanies alcoholism. Degenerative changes in the diencephalon, particularly the hippocampus, are seen at autopsy. It is possible that a patient with repeated blackouts eventually goes on to develop the Wernicke-Korsakoff array of symptoms. If so, is it possible that high-dose vitamin B therapy may prevent or attenuate blackouts?

It might be assumed that those who sustain a complete loss of memory for hours or days would be sufficiently frightened to discontinue using the substance that caused the deficit. Unfortunately, blackouts only infrequently result in abstinence. Individuals who experience multiple amnesias seem to accept them as the price paid for intoxication, and they equate them with the memory loss that accompanies passing out. These are completely different conditions. Passing out is associated with the inability to function actively. During a blackout, people can still perform, appear normal, and as we shall see, become a hazard to themselves and others.

DIFFERENTIAL DIAGNOSIS

Not everyone who experiences a memory loss during alcohol intoxication has a blackout. Any disruption of the hippocampal complex can evoke an amnestic response. The Wernicke-Korsakoff syndrome has been mentioned. Certain head traumas (the postconcussion syndrome), or hypoxia of the brain as in carbon monoxide poisoning may sometimes present a similar picture.

Simulating amnesia by malingering in order to try to evade responsibility for some act must be considered. The amnesias that accompany delirium or coma are readily differentiated because of the profound alterations of consciousness. Psychogenic amnesias occur preponderantly during war or natural disasters as a part of a severe stress syndrome. They may also take place during catastrophic events involving one or a small number of people. Memories blacked out by severe stress are often retrievable under dissociating agents like hypnosis or sodium pentothal, differentiating them from blackouts.

LEGAL SIGNIFICANCE

Blackouts assume a legal importance when some major accident or crime occurs, and the accused had been intoxicated at the time of the incident. The individual may disclaim any knowledge of the accident, assault, or homicide and of the events leading up to and subsequent to it. Whether such a person is capable of premeditating a crime and whether the capacity to understand the nature of the criminal act is present, are questions posed to expert witnesses.

Proof of whether the accused was actually in an amnesic state is also sought. Amnesia is not a defense against the accusation of a criminal act, but it may show diminished capacity and result in a less severe sentence. Various states handle the diminished capacity defense differently.

Wolf has recently reported on five young, alcoholic, Alaskan natives each of whom committed a homicide during one of their many blackouts. During experimentally induced alcohol intoxications while in jail, the subjects were unable to recall the homicide or other incidents temporally related to the crime.

They blacked out during the alcohol intoxication test, and the author noticed an abrupt mood change that seemed to coincide with the amnesic episode. The mood shifted from enjoyment to anger, at times associated with overt, violent behavior. The prisoners later remembered their alcoholic exposure as pleasurable because of the lack of recall of the dysphoric mood interval.

Suicide attempts have been reported in connection with blackouts. These are believed to be related to the depressive mood that may occur, the disinhibited loss of control over behavior, and the retention of the physical capability to execute the suicidal effort.

SUMMARY

The presence of a global amnesia for hours or days during and after the liberal usage of alcoholic beverages is an interesting event. That a person without a major disruption of consciousness is unable to remember what happened must be impressive, but apparently most drinkers learn to tolerate such lapses. Serious adverse consequences are possible during the amnestic episode because mood changes and disinhibited behavior can accompany the loss of the ability to lay down recently acquired information. At times physicians will be called upon to testify on the nature, the cause, and the differential diagnosis of a blackout when a criminal act has been committed and the alleged assailant has no recall for the incident.

Blackouts must have a biochemical substrate that would be worth knowing so that our understanding of the process is improved. Furthermore, their prevention might be possible. Since they are fairly well reproduced in those drinkers who routinely experience them, the more thorough study of the alcohol amnestic state is both possible and justifiable. It may also be worthwhile to follow a group of people vulnerable to blackouts in order to determine whether the amnestic-confabulatory syndrome occurs with greater frequency with them than with other alcoholics.

BIBLIOGRAPHY

- Goodwin, D.W. Alcoholic blackout and how to prevent it. In: I.M. Burnbaum and E.S. Parker, eds. *Alcohol and Human Memory*. Lawrence Erlbaum Assoc. Hillsdale, N.J. 1977.
- Goodwin, D.W. et al. Alcoholic blackouts and Korsakoff's syndrome. In: M. Gross, Ed. *Alcohol Intoxication and Withdrawal II*. Plenum, New York, 1975.
- Ryback, R.S. The continuum and specificity of the effects of alcohol on memory. Quart. J. Stud. Alcohol. 32:995-1061, 1971.
- Tamarin, J.S. et al. Alcohol and memory: Amnesia and short-term memory function during experimentally induced intoxication. Am. J. Psychiatry. 127:95-100, 1971.
- Tarter, R.E. and Schneider, D.V. Blackouts: Relationship with memory capacity and alcoholism history. Arch. Gen. Psychiat. 33: 1492-1946, 1976.
- Tarter, R.E. and Sugerman, A.A. Craving for alcohol. In: M.M. Gross, ed. *Alcohol Intoxication and Withdrawal IIIb*. Plenum, New York, 1977.
- Wolf, A.S. Homicide and blackout in Alaskan natives. J. Stud. Alcohol, 41: 456-462, 1980.

18. Pathological Intoxication

Pathological intoxication, or alcohol idiosyncratic intoxication as it is called in DSM III, is a rather infrequent condition. But when a case is seen, it remains in the memory of those nearby because of the impressive panic or rage reactions. An older name for the disorder is *mania á potu.* This term should be discarded because it has also been used in connection with the delirium tremens.

CLINICAL FEATURES

The essential characteristic is a marked behavioral change, usually in the direction of inappropriate belligerence and assaultiveness following the ingestion of a small quantity of alcoholic beverages. The amount consumed may be as little as one drink, but sometimes larger amounts are required to evoke the condition. However, it is not a quantity sufficient to produce intoxication. The behavior represents a marked change from the person's usual comportment.

The mental state reflects the unpredictable and destructive behavioral pattern. Confusion and disorganization of thought processes are evident. Speech is either incoherent or based on delusional thinking. It is the explosive fury in connection with the consumption of less than intoxicating amounts of alcohol that is most impressive. The rage reaction can result in serious injury to relatives, friends, or strangers. Homicides are a possibility and a few serious suicide attempts have been reported. The condition terminates in a deep sleep. Upon awakening a total or partial amnesia for the episode is present.

DOES IT EXIST?

A number of investigators of this problem do not believe that pathological intoxication exists as an entity separable from other disorders. They argue that the unpredictable violent episodes represent dissociation states in which the alcohol drunk is incidental. Going berserk can happen to anyone under maximal stress whose ability to cope with the enormous pressures has collapsed. Running amok and negi negi are acting out syndromes in primitive societies that are related to the taboo of expressing strong personal feelings. They include impulsive, aimless destructiveness terminating in claims of amnesia. Even in the developed countries unmotivated outbursts of hostile activities are becoming more common. Acute paranoid psychotic reactions are usually considered responsible for these aberrations. A number of patients with temporal lobe dysrhythmias manifest aggressiveness, hyperactivity, and deluded behavior. Genetic forms of sudden, unexpected violence are also described.

In recent years the picture of abrupt, unthinking harm to one's self or others followed by an amnestic episode may be caused by drugs other than ethanol. Phencyclidine toxicity can precisely duplicate what we understand as pathological intoxication. Acute amphetamine or cocaine psychosis is another condition that would have to be considered. Barbiturates and similarly acting brain depressants are capable of inducing abrupt, assaultive outbursts. So a person who has taken a drink and had a rage reaction may have other important psychoactive drugs in his or her system.

Acute alcohol intoxication is known to be associated with purposeless violence, stuporousness, and amnesia. But if the diagnosis of pathologic intoxication has any reason for existence as a discrete entity, it is in the hypersensitivity of a few people to modest, nonintoxicating amounts. Therefore, many unrelated behavioral disturbances have been misdiagnosed as pathological intoxication. This does not mean that the condition is nonexistent. It means that it is not a frequent syndrome.

CRITERIA FOR THE DIAGNOSIS
OF PATHOLOGICAL INTOXICATION

Although rather rare, instances of pathological intoxication do occur. It is neither difficult nor improper to make such a diagnosis under the following conditions.

1. The person either has never used alcohol previously or has had a normal response to it in the past.

2. An insult to the brain, usually a substantial head injury or encephalitis has taken place. Some students of the condition have suggested that preexisting epilepsy, or unstable, hysterical personality or cerebral arteriosclerosis may predispose to the pathological response to alcohol. Others have emphasized that severe levels of stress are of paramount importance in precipitating pathological intoxication. Even hypoglycemia has been sus-

pected, but not proven, in a few cases. Perhaps, the common denominator to all of the alleged contributory causes is impairment of cerebral nutrition or damage or death of specific inhibitory neurones.

3. Following recovery from the head trauma or other disorder the person loses his or her tolerance to alcohol. He or she responds unthinkingly, impulsively, and belligerently to no or minor provocation after consuming alcohol. The amount may be as little as one or two ounces of ethanol. In order to make a secure diagnosis of pathological intoxication, a blood alcohol concentration of less than 0.1 percent would seem necessary. Otherwise pathological intoxication could not be differentiated from alcohol intoxication with an associated rage response.

4. A challenge with the same amount of alcohol reproduces the explosive behavior. It is preferable to give the drug intravenously so that the patient is unaware when the alcohol is instilled. Sometimes attempts to reproduce the noxious behavior will not succeed in a neutral or benign environment. Whether the deliberate introduction of a stressor should be tried might be considered. Precautionary restraints may be indicated. A history of repeated, bizarre spontaneous episodes following the moderate use of alcohol would favor the diagnosis.

5. Following the outburst which may be brief or last for hours, a period of exhaustion and sleep intervenes. Upon awakening, the individual cannot remember the unusual events in which he or she was involved.

6. The offensive behavior should be atypical of the person's conduct when not drinking.

THE INTERACTION OF BRAIN DAMAGE AND ALCOHOL

It is well known that posttraumatic encephalopathy alone can be accompanied by unprovoked assaultiveness. A sudden burst of assaultive behavior following little or no provocation can be seen in those who have sustained cerebral damage from many causes, especially trauma.

High levels of alcohol intake are a major cause of criminal, aggressive acts in this society. Drunkenness produces impaired judgment, reduction of controls over behavior, and paranoid misinterpretation of the environment. The result can be an alcohol provoked rage.

Since both brain damage and alcohol themselves are capable of producing seriously aberrant behaviors, it is hardly surprising that the combination will do likewise. In the person who is susceptible to pathological intoxication the brain damaged person requires the triggering action of small quantities of alcohol to unleash the hostility and its sequellae.

Pathological intoxication, therefore, exists as a narrow band on the continuum between the spontaneous violence of some brain damaged people and the overtly aggressive acts of those who lose control under the influence of large amounts of ethanol. A belief in its existence is justified because of people whose conduct disorders will be brought under control by complete abstinence from "social" amounts of beverage alcohol exist.

LOSS OF TOLERANCE TO ALCOHOL

Since pathological intoxication represents a serious loss of the ability to ingest alcohol, it may be useful to mention other circumstances in which tolerance to this substance is also diminished. People who have sustained previous head injuries may describe a loss of ability to "hold their liquor" even when the changes do not include hostile displays. Such individuals tend to pass out after a few drinks.

Usually, aging brings with it a diminution of tolerance. This is presumably due to a loss of the brain's ability to compensate for the psychomotor changes that accompany the intoxicated state. No doubt the impaired metabolism of alcohol also contributes to the inability to deal with alcohol as well as during the younger years.

Naturally, people who stop sustained drinking practices will notice an increased sensitivity to lesser amounts when they resume drinking again. It is generally believed that unusually fatigued persons or those with debilitating illnesses will be more affected by alcohol than was customary for them.

Liver damage severe enough to interfere with the enzyme systems that metabolize alcohol or acetaldehyde will have blood and brain alcohol levels much higher than estimated in consideration of the quantity imbibed. End-stage alcoholics without cirrhosis can lose some of their tolerance. This is ascribed to the diffuse brain damage resulting from chronic alcoholism.

FORENSIC ASPECTS

Criminal acts committed under circumstances in which pathological intoxication might be postulated represent an important defense of a person accused of an act of violence. The consumption of large amounts of alcohol might be a mitigating factor insofar as intent is concerned, when a major crime is executed. But if pathological intoxication can be proven, it may more readily constitute grounds for a verdict of involuntary manslaughter in a case of a homicide. This is especially true if the pathological violence were the first instance of such behavior. The defense may be invalidated if the defendant knows that he or she is prone to automatic violent deeds if he or she takes small amounts of alcohol.

The diagnosis of pathological intoxication is not easily made. A detailed case study must be done and the six criteria noted above substantially satisfied. One important differential diagnostic possibility must be excluded: malingering. Naturally, when the threat of punishment is anticipated, a lack of recall for the violent incident might be claimed. Inconsistencies in the story must be carefully sought for. Polygraph tests, even the willingness to take such tests, may be helpful in forming a personal opinion even if such testing is not admissible evidence in court.

DISCUSSION

The literature on pathological intoxication is quite confusing. A wide variety of bellicose disturbances that happen to occur in connection with drinking are randomly grouped together by some clinicians as pathological intoxication. These include psychomotor epilepsy, delirium tremens, violence resulting from drunkenness, and certain dissociation states.

Unfortunately, no reliable objective test is available to support the diagnosis. The recurrence of assaultive behavior under test conditions is supportive of the diagnosis when it occurs, but negative tests do not necessarily rule out the condition. Temporal lobe spiking on the electroencephalogram following the ingestion of small amounts of alcohol occurs only in a small percentage of these people.

Nevertheless, it is believed that this condition represents a rare, but real diagnostic entity that can be sorted out from the other states mentioned. This opinion is held on the basis of clinical impressions of a small number of cases, seen over the years, that conformed to the criteria mentioned here.

The mechanism of the loss of tolerance to alcohol in pathological intoxication would be worth investigating. Both tissue and behavioral intolerance may play a role. Tissue intolerance would result from impaired neurones being less able to withstand the toxic effect of alcohol. Behavioral loss of tolerance signifies that the adaptive and monitoring functions of the brain are diminished to the point that antisocial impulses cannot be controlled or modulated, and they come forth as impulsive, maladaptive behaviors.

BIBLIOGRAPHY

- Bach-Y-Rita, G., Lion, J.R. and Ervin, F.R. Pathological intoxication and electroencephalographic status. Amer. J. Psychiat. 127: 698-702, 1970.

- Coid, J. *Mania á potu:* A critical review of pathological intoxication. Psychological Med. 9: 709-719, 1979.
- Hollender, M.H. Pathological intoxication—Is there such an entity? J. Clin. Psychiat. 40: 424-426, 1979.
- Kosbab, F.P. and Kuhnley, E.J. Pathological intoxication. Psychiat. Opinion. 15: 35-38, 1978.
- Maletsky, B.M. The diagnosis of pathological intoxication. J. Studies Alcohol. 37: 1215-1228, 1976.

19. The One-Vehicle Accident

If you are becoming concerned about the increasing number of homicides, consider that more fatal injuries result from traffic accidents each year than from homicides and suicides combined.

Many young Americans lost their lives during the Vietnam conflict, but many more lost their lives during those same years in domestic traffic accidents. It is incomprehensible why so few people become upset about the 45,000 or so who are killed and the hundreds of thousands who are injured in motor vehicle accidents each year. More than a third of these injuries and a half of the deaths are alcohol-related. With wisdom and desire, many of these casualties could be prevented.

THE SINGLE-VEHICLE ACCIDENT (SVA)

The single-vehicle accident is a special type of car accident, and one in which alcohol and, to a lesser extent, drugs play a significant role. In various studies 18 to 51 percent of drivers involved in multivehicle fatalities had a blood alcohol concentration of 0.1 percent or higher.

As many as 41 to 72 percent of the drivers in single-car fatalities had BACs in that range. These figures are compiled from 12 studies of multivehicular accidents and 17 studies of one-car accidents.

The statistics from a number of states reveal that the long-term trend in SVA fatalities as compared with all auto accidents is upward. In 1951, 25 percent of all automobile deaths were one-car crashes. By 1961 the percentage had risen to 39.6 percent. In 1977 the majority (56 percent) of fatal car accidents were SVAs.

During the last year for which data are available, 1980, the percentage was 61. Therefore the SVA has surpassed the multiple-car accident as a fatal casualty-producing agent, and its association with intoxication is unquestioned.

Of course, alcohol is not involved in all SVAs. From the table it can be seen that other causes exist. However, in 40 to 60 percent of such mishaps alcohol intoxication and related effects contribute to the accident. It is evident

111

Table 19–1
Single-Vehicle Accident Causes

Driver Failure
Driver intoxication (alcohol or drugs or both)
Sleepiness
Excessive speed
Inept driving skills
Operator distraction
Illness (pain, stupor, syncope, seizure)
Impaired visual or auditory acuity
Suicide attempt

Vehicle Failure
Tire blowout
Brake failure
Accelerator jam

Hazardous Driving Conditions
Dangerous roadway
Adverse weather conditions
Sun or headlight glare
Obstacle on road

that most of the SVA causes listed under "Driver Failure" can be attributed to intoxication by some substance.

SVAs tend to occur late at night or on weekends, coinciding with the periods of heavier drinking and fatigue. Frequently, multiple causes are involved in the crash. A speeding drunk driver dozes at the wheel and cannot react quickly enough to prevent a crash. The results of an SVA may be vehicle overturn; car leaving the roadway, striking an object, driving into a ditch, other car, body of water, or embankment; or a collision with some moving object such as a pedestrian, a cyclist, vehicle, or train.

The role of alcohol in SVAs is obvious. In amounts as low as 0.04 percent (one to two drinks) some mild decrement in psychomotor performance is measurable. The impairment increases in a linear fashion until BACs are reached that are incompatible with the ability to attempt to drive. It is believed that SVAs are more serious than multicar accidents because higher speeds are recorded in the former type of accident.

SUICIDE

Suicide has special relationships both with SVAs and with alcohol. People intent on suicide have been known to employ their cars to achieve this end.

The self-destructive drives may come forth during drinking bouts, or may have existed prior to it, and the individuals used alcohol to reduce their fears and to benumb themselves.

One estimate suggests that 10 to 15 percent of SVAs have a suicidal intent, although this figure has been disputed as too high by others. It has been found that an unusually large number of holders of double indemnity policies die in SVAs.

A recent report from England indicates that suicide is not a frequent cause of single-car, single-occupant deaths. The highest number of such deaths occurred in the 14- to 34-year age group whereas the suicide distribution increases with age. The age of drivers who died alone in their vehicles was the same as those in SVAs with other passengers.

The authors concluded that undoubtedly a few single-car, single-occupant accidents were intentional deaths, but the numbers were not large enough to affect the reported suicide rate. Therefore, disguised suicides of this sort do not represent a major contribution to the causes of SVAs.

EPIDEMIOLOGY

From the available information it is possible to separate two distinct but overlapping drinking-driving populations: the SVA drivers and the multivehicle accident drivers.

Those involved in SVAs are younger, often in their teens or twenties. The age group at greatest risk are those between 14 and 24. The youthfulness of these drivers implies an inexperience with driving or drinking or both. Another rise in the curve is seen among elderly drivers. Adults between the ages of 25 and 55 have the lowest rates. SVA drivers are likely to be single, separated, or widowed males.

The youthful SVA driver is often characterized as having socially deviant traits as manifested by callousness, hedonism, emotional immaturity, irresponsibility, poor judgment, and the ability to rationalize his or her destructive behavior as warranted, reasonable, and justified. These personality attributes are sometimes associated with youthfulness, and intoxication tends to exacerbate impulsive, risk-taking behavior.

The fact that a surprising number of SVAs happen during fair weather conditions on straight roads within close proximity to the operator's home indicates that driver failure, rather than the adverse nondriver factors, are the important causative elements. It has been found that most of the dead SVA drivers had not used seatbelts.

BLOOD ALCOHOL LEVELS

The high percentage of SVA drivers who had BACs over 0.10 percent has been mentioned. In addition, the average BAC for this group is significantly higher than for the multicar accident group. Drivers between the ages of 40 and 60 had the highest BACs, but they accounted for fewer SVAs.

This negative correlation might indicate that age-related factors such as inexperience or recklessness were more important than the degree of intoxication. An equally plausible assumption is that the middle-aged drivers may have acquired some measure of tolerance to the effects of alcohol by regular drinking and were less impaired by it.

SPEEDING

More than half of the SVAs occurred at excessive speeds. The median speed recorded was between 50 and 60 miles an hour. In contrast, multivehicular accidents were most frequently recorded at 40 to 50 miles an hour. Despite the higher speeds, most SVAs took place on roads with lower speed limits than the multivehicular accidents did.

SINGLE VS. MULTIPLE OCCUPANCY

The solitary driver is more likely to become involved in an SVA than the accompanied one. This may be due to the restraining effects of the other occupants upon obviously unsafe driving practices. Uncertainty exists in the literature regarding accidents involving one or multiple occupants in an SVA. One report cites a 2½ times greater frequency of unaccompanied over accompanied drivers. In a study of 15- to 19-year-olds in SVAs, only one-quarter occurred when the driver was the sole occupant of the car. Obviously, more information is needed.

SUMMARY

The single-vehicle accident is becoming an increasingly important cause of autocide, injury, and destruction. It now accounts for a majority of motor vehicle deaths. Alcohol is an important factor in these crashes. Youthful drivers are at particular risk. By far, most one-car accidents result from driver failure. Therefore, preventive strategies must include efforts to change the driving behavior of the drinker.

When it becomes generally understood that consumption of even social amounts of alcoholic beverages causes some impairment of driving skills, perhaps fewer drinkers will drive. Consistent and stringent enforcement policies equitably carried out will discourage others who persist in driving after imbibing. Whether raising the drinking and/or the driving age would make a significant impact should be studied.

BIBLIOGRAPHY

- Huffine, C.L. Equivocal single auto fatal traffic accidents. Life Threatening Behavior 1:83-95, 1971.
- Jenkins, J. and Salisbury, P. Single car road deaths—disguised suicides? British Med. J. 281:1041, 1980.
- Krantz, P. Differences between single and multiple automobile fatal accidents. Accid. Anal. & Prev. 1:225-236, 1979.
- Schmidt, C.M. Suicide by vehicular crash. Am. J. Psychiat. 134:175-178, 1977.
- Technical Support Document. Third Special Report to the U.S. Congress on Alcohol and Health. U.S. Government Printing Office, Washington, D.C. 20402, 1978. Stock No. 017-024-00892-3.

20. Alcohol-Related Disorders: Early Identification

Many aspects of the 1980 presidential race were unusual, but in one respect it was unique. Never before have four of the leading candidates or quasi-candidates had close relatives who have publicly acknowledged that they had been in trouble with alcohol.

Betty Ford, Billy Carter, Joy Baker, and Joan Kennedy have made frank statements about their drinking problems and their treatment experiences. Many other prominent politicians, executives, sports figures, and entertainers have recently come forth and announced similar difficulties.

It is heartening to see that the symbolic closet where alcoholics have traditionally secluded themselves is now ajar, and that those in need of help are seeking it at an earlier phase of their drinking careers. Healthy cultural shifts appear to be under way that will provide an opportunity for the earlier diagnosis and treatment of problem drinkers.

Health professionals must prepare themselves for the new situation, sharpening their diagnostic skills, detecting early dysfunctional drinking, and developing effective techniques for motivating and managing the pre-alcoholic. In an effort to detect the premonitory signs and symptoms of dysfunctional drinking, a review of the danger signals is attempted here. In general these are signals, not diagnostic certainties. They are intended to arouse suspicion that the patient may be at risk of impairing himself or herself if drinking continues at the current level. The signals to be mentioned are medical indicators. Very often behavioral and interpersonal danger signs coexist.

THE "HITTING BOTTOM" NOTION

Many individuals and groups, including AA, have espoused the belief that before drinkers can really be driven to begin the recovery process they must "hit bottom." This means that their health is severely impaired, family situation wrecked, finances depleted, or self-respect shattered. Only then can they mobilize sufficient willpower to start the long, hard road back to sobriety and rehabilitation. Short of "hitting bottom," rationalizations that they can stop drinking whenever they want to, or that their misfortunes are not really due to excessive drinking, may persist.

For some, it may be necessary to be confronted with a total personal disaster before sufficient resolve to finally stop using alcohol is achieved. On the other hand, this critical point may occur too late. By then brain damage may be irreparable, liver failure irreversible, or the social situation may be irretrievable.

Therefore early case finding and entry into treatment during mid-level drinking careers rather than during the final stages is where our present efforts should be directed. Mid-level drinking disorders are more difficult to identify and are at a phase when it is harder to persuade the patient of the need to make major changes in his or her life. The conventional treatment methods may not be appropriate for these incipient alcoholics and improved or alternative measures may have to be employed.

ALCOHOL-RELATED DISEASES OR SYMPTOMS

A sizable number of disorders are directly or indirectly associated with injudicious alcohol consumption. These abnormalities are not invariably associated with alcohol, but their presence should raise the possibility of that etiology. Furthermore, like intoxication or hangover, the frequency, not the existence of these events, will determine the degree of risk of impending alcoholism.

Alcoholic Fatty Liver, Pancreatitis, and Gastritis

A smooth, non-tender enlargement of the liver with or without abnormal liver function tests in connection with drinking episodes is evidence of higher levels of ethanol intake than the liver cells can successfully metabolize. Severe, constant upper abdominal pain and tenderness usually radiating to the back reflects pancreatic inflammation and that too many years of excessive drinking already have occurred. Anorexia, nausea, and vomiting, sometimes bloody, is evidence of a direct toxic effect of alcohol on the stomach lining with associated erosions or ulcerations.

Poor Nutrition and Immune Response

In addition to an inattention to proper nutrition and hygienic measures, a preoccupation with drinking will cause a variety of pulmonary infections from aspiration while drunk, to a failure of the normal pulmonary immune defense mechanisms.

Impaired absorption of nutrients and vitamins, particularly thiamine, and changes in intestinal motility contribute to the diarrhea that sometimes accompanies drinking bouts. Many other nutritional deficiencies can be identified.

Neurologic Changes

An increased patellar reflex has been noted in alcohol abusers. The earliest signs of peripheral neuropathy would include somewhat diminished touch, temperature, pain, and position sensations. Atrophy and pain of the calf muscles have been described by a few authors early in the course of excessive drinking.

Hematologic Abnormalities

A number of hematologic changes can occur caused by a variety of alcohol-related disturbances. These include a folate deficiency producing megaloblastosis or macrocytosis detectable in an elevated mean corpuscular volume. Pyridoxine deficiency can result in a sideroblastic anemia. Obscure instances of thrombocytopenia and bleeding may be traced to alcohol overuse.

Myopathy

Lower extremity muscle aches, weakness, cramping, and tenderness may be symptoms of alcoholic myopathy, and these can occur rather early in the evolution of the drinking career. Cardiomyopathy, on the other hand, is a late evidence of alcoholism.

The Skin and Alcohol

Long before rhinophyma, acne rosacea, and spider nevi make their appearance, less obvious alterations of the skin become noticeable. The face may be puffy, the cheeks and nose flushed, and the conjunctival vessels injected. The tongue is smooth and red (except when it is coated with chlorophyll) reflecting a vitamin B deficiency. Palmar erythema may be visible before cirrhosis can be diagnosed.

Cigarette burns between the index and middle fingers or on the chest, and contusions and bruises should be considered suspicious of alcoholic stupor and injury. Insect bites and frostbite are some of the hazards of spending a night out-of-doors in an alcoholic coma.

Blackouts

Loss of recall for a period of time when the drinker was apparently conscious and functioning well is not always a tardive sign of alcoholism. Amnesia for the hours or days of a drinking bout may occur shortly after heavy drinking has commenced and tends to recur during subsequent sprees.

Impotence and Loss of Libido

Male impotence can be an acute or a chronic consequence of considerable drinking. Alcohol appears to block the synthesis of testosterone in the gonads while accelerating its breakdown in the liver. Libido decrease is a somewhat later symptom resulting from low levels of testosterone availability, or to its conversion to estrogen-like substances.

Cancer and Alcohol

Drinking alcoholic beverages leads to an increased risk of cancer at various sites of the body. Heavy drinking is associated with an increased probability of developing cancers of the tongue, mouth, pharynx, larynx, esophagus, and liver. Heavy alcohol and tobacco use act synergistically to increase the rate of head and neck cancers. While alcohol is not a carcinogen, it may either act as a cocarcinogen or as a solvent for cancer-producing polyaromatic hydrocarbons.

LABORATORY AIDS IN THE DIAGNOSIS OF IMPENDING ALCOHOLISM

The demonstration of a positive blood alcohol and blood acetaldehyde during or shortly after drinking is not a valuable prognostic indicator of impending alcoholism. One possible exception is elevated blood alcohol levels associated with fairly normal behavior. It might indicate high levels of tolerance. (See also the criteria used by Morse and Hurt listed in References.)

An elevated blood lactate simply reflects the shift from pyruvate to lactate metabolism. Lactic acidosis, however, decreases uric acid excretion and results in hyperuricemia or even attacks of gout. These latter findings are suspicious of but not confirmatory of excessive use of ethanol.

Selected individuals may show a rise in serum triglycerides shortly after alcohol use. Such elevations return to normal within two weeks of abstinence. The very low density lipoproteins and chylomicrons are elevated and may remain high if alcohol is used chronically. When severe liver damage supervenes, plasma lipid levels will fall below normal because of an inability of the liver to synthesize lipoproteins.

Alcoholic acidosis and ketosis in the absence of diabetes, especially if accompanied by urinary ketone bodies, are suggestive of recent heavy binge-type drinking.

A very low blood sugar in a heavy drinker suggests that glycogen stores are exhausted, and alcohol metabolism is preventing gluconeogenesis from fat and amino acids. Since hypoglycemia has many causes, it is not diagnostic of alcohol excess, but it should always be considered in instances of coma in someone with alcohol on the breath.

Serum gamma-glutamyl transpeptidase (GGT) is elevated in drinkers who may have little evidence of hepatic malfunction. Although it gradually decreases during the abstinent period, it may remain elevated for weeks after cessation of heavy drinking. It may serve as a useful screening test for patients entering a medical care unit for reasons other than an alcohol problem. It is not completely specific for alcoholic liver dysfunction. An elevated GGT in the absence of barbiturate use or biliary disease is good supportive evidence for dysfunctional drinking and should be so considered by the physician and the patient.

Serum glutamic oxalacetic transaminase (SGOT), serum glutamic pyruvic transaminase (SGPT), lactic dehydrogenase (LDH), and similar enzymatic tests are all nonspecific in that they are elevated in response to muscle injury, use of certain drugs, acute liver and kidney damage, etc. The GGT is fairly specific for liver damage or barbiturate use. It is, perhaps, most useful for alcoholic liver impairment, remaining elevated after the other enzyme tests have reverted to normal.

Low folic acid, thiamine, and phosphate levels have been reported in abstinent alcoholic patients, and these might be considered supportive of a diagnosis of excessive drinking.

Efforts to develop empirical markers of alcoholism, for example, the alpha-aminobutyric acid to leucine ratio, have not yet been refined to the point where they are clinically feasible.

In an important article Morse and Hurt[1] summarize their use of laboratory findings in alcohol problems. They consider a patient to be an alcoholic if he or she comes in for a general examination with a blood alcohol level of more than 100 mg/dl, if the BAL is 150 mg/dl without signs of intoxication, or if a BAL of 300 mg/dl is obtained at any time. Sixty-three percent of patients admitted to the alcoholism unit at Mayo Clinic had an elevated GGT. The SGOT was abnormal in 48 percent, and macrocytosis as measured by the mean corpuscular volume was abnormal in 26 percent. Serum triglycerides were elevated in 22 percent, alkaline phosphotase in 16 percent, serum bilirubin in 13 percent, and serum uric acid in 10 percent.

A recent development has been the combined use of the SMAV12, the

SMAV6, and the complete blood count as a method for establishing a diagnosis of early alcoholism. These tests are routinely requested and do not add to patient costs. Utilizing this battery of 25 tests and applying a quadratic discriminant analysis to the data, Ryback et al.[2] were able to predict 94 percent of alcoholics in treatment programs and 100 percent of nonalcoholics correctly. Sixteen of 23 alleged nonalcoholics who drank more than three drinks a day were also found to give positive results. The test was not accurate for those over 65 years of age. When the statistical software for the test becomes available, it may become a valuable screening device in physicians' offices and hospital admission services.

SUMMARY

Assuredly, many patients with suspicious physical or laboratory evidence of incipient alcoholism will refuse to act on this information. Nevertheless, they should be informed of their situation as they would be in the early stages of any illness that is detected.

Some patients will take appropriate corrective action on their own or with the assistance of a therapist. Early identification and intervention are possible and, with skilled treatment, will be more rewarding than caring for chronic, end-stage alcoholics.

REFERENCES

1. Morse, R. M. and Hurt, R. D. Screening for alcoholism. JAMA 242: 2688-2690, 1979.
2. Ryback, R. S., Eckardt, M. J. and Pautler, C. P. Biochemical and hematological correlates of alcoholism. Research Communications in Chemistry, Pathology and Pharmacology, 27: 533-550, 1980.

21. How to Become an Alcoholic

With 10 percent of the drinking population having problems managing their drinking, it may seem superfluous to provide instructions on how to become an alcoholic. It apparently is an almost inevitable process for millions of our citizens. The point, of course, is that by learning of the techniques of drinking destructively, someone might use the information in order to avoid such practices. In this chapter alcoholism is used to include both problem drinking and alcoholic addiction.

IN THE BEGINNING

A certain amount of the loading in favor of becoming alcoholic apparently happens when a certain sperm cell fertilizes a certain egg cell. The studies in which identical twins were raised either by their natural or adoptive parents indicate that inherited factors do have some impact upon subsequent drinking practices.

Identical twins, one raised by the natural alcoholic parents and one by adoptive, nonalcoholic parents, will have similar rates of alcohol-related disorders. When an identical twin of nonalcoholic parents is raised by alcoholic adoptive parents—one or both—the chances of that twin becoming alcoholic are approximately the same as the twin raised by the biologic parents.

How strong are these factors in determining whether a child will become an alcoholic? Not very great. Although one or both parents may have been considered to be alcoholics, neither may have possessed the genetic predisposition. Even if a child has inherited the genetic component, it amounts to no more than a vulnerability to becoming an alcoholic. Therefore, children of families with numbers of inordinate drinkers have a responsibility to themselves to be particularly careful about using alcoholic beverages. Whether it is, indeed, a genetically determined effect in any specific child is unknown. It is just as likely to be an acquired family tradition to drink excessively. In both instances dangerous drinking practices can be avoided by being aware of the vulnerability. To slip into the family's pattern has only one advantage. One can always blame it on one's chromosomes.

THE MILIEU

Much more important than heredity are the environmental impacts—the strong conditioning one acquires from relatives, friends, peer groups, media, educators, pastors, and others about how to deal with life stress and how to drink.

It is possible for some young people to wind up as adult alcoholics by being either neglected or overprotected during their early growing-up period. Neglect deprives the child of suitable role models to emulate. Learning how to relate to other people, a process that should begin within the family group, takes place elsewhere or not at all. Noncaring parents surrender the training of the youngster to anyone or any group that happens to be in contact with the child rather than a devoted family unit. Neglect deprives the child of needed supports in time of crisis.

Overprotection is equally detrimental. Independence, self-esteem, and problem-solving and decision-making abilities are not acquired. The maturational process atrophies. The child's ability to endure difficult experiences, loss, frustration, and defeat remains undeveloped. In other words the immaturity imposed upon the young person helps to shape alcohol-consuming behavior and in fact, many other undesirable adult behaviors.

We are not sure of what an ideal upbringing consists of, but certain features of the parent-child interaction like love, trust, consistency, concern—not overconcern—willingness to permit the child to assume responsibilities, and a relationship that permits the discussion of problems, are certainly components of a helpful atmosphere in which to grow up.

ON BECOMING AN ALCOHOLIC

One way to get into trouble with drinking is being able to hold your liquor better than most people. Unfortunately, folk knowledge assumes the opposite. But being able to consume unusually large quantities before becoming affected by it, simply means that the body is exposed to and must deal with the inordinate amounts being poured in. The ability to remain relatively sober while others slide under the table, unable to drink more, may be due either to the development of tolerance after consistent exposure to ethanol, being a very large person (because alcohol diffuses uniformly into all cells), or having some metabolic facility in dealing with the chemical.

Regarding resistance to the intoxicating effects of liquor, a vivid description of Jack London's ability to handle alcoholic beverages can be found in his memoirs "John Barleycorn."* London died at age 40, a suicide with advanced alcoholic hepatitis and nephritis. He discovered his amazing ability to drink long and hard without passing out as a child. He never liked the taste of booze, but drunkenness was the social norm on the San Francisco Bay waterfront of the day, and he worked hard achieving a rousing intoxication whenever his friends and the bars were available.

But there are many other ways to become an alcoholic, and some of them should be mentioned. Denial and rationalization are two psychological techniques used to avoid the reality of impending or existing trouble with one's drinking. When the consequences of drinking are disastrous—job losses, arrests, family problems, car accidents, and so forth—these are often considered reasons to drink rather than reasons to terminate one's drinking. This sort of evasion of the reality situation is a common way to become a confirmed alcoholic.

Certain health problems are alcohol-related. Specific kinds of liver damage, pancreatitis, gastritis, and in the later stages, neuritis, esophageal varicosities, and other ailments are evidence that the body is not successfully handling the amount of alcohol imbibed. Obviously, a decision has to be made about drinking, but all too often it is either abrogated, or the physical distress itself becomes a reason to drink more.

Many people drink because of unease, anxiety, and depression. For example, "drowning one's sorrows" is an everyday expression. Alcohol may erase these noxious feelings, but it is well documented that as one continues to imbibe, tension and anxiety levels rise again. Furthermore, the morning-after state is often quite unpleasant. Therefore, something is needed to ease the psychological and physical unpleasantness. Alcohol reverses the miserable feelings, but it may produce an endless cycle of dysphoria → drinking → dysphoria → drinking.

The positive rewards of moderate drinking are not to be ignored since they involve 90 percent of all users of beverage alcohol, the nonproblem drinkers. Tension relaxation, a smoothing out of interpersonal irritants, perhaps a distancing from the immediacy of life's travails are some of the positive reinforcers of small amounts of ethanol.

Repeated loss of control over drinking, however, is an ominous sign for the consumer. Successful social drinkers use certain cues that tell them when to stop. It may be a matter of counting the number of drinks or drinking only during specific social occasions. Maintenance of control may also be managed by an internal feedback mechanism that estimates how high one feels or

---

John Barleycorn: Alcoholic Memoirs by Jack London. Reprinted by Robert Bentley, Cambridge, Mass. 02139, 1964.

whether any signs of incoordination or slurring of speech are perceptible. These become stop signals for the modest drinker. People who are unaware of or who deliberately ignore these internal or external warning cues are at risk of overdrinking even when they have no intention of doing so.

Counseling certain alcoholics includes learning the stop signals and learning how to respond to them. A few chronic alcoholics demonstrate another sort of loss of control. A single drink precipitates a drinking spree. They appear unable to stop once primed by a small amount of alcohol. People with problems of loss of control must either abstain completely, learn strategies of maintaining control, or accept inevitable alcoholism.

Mental attitudes toward the symbolic meaning of drinking may trap some people into a career of excessive consumption, culminating in alcoholism. The notion that drinking a lot is macho, or that, as in the case of young people, being intoxicated is manly, can lead to precarious drinking patterns. Naturally, this sort of symbolism is used in media advertising extensively. One can hardly watch television, listen to the radio, or read newspapers or magazines without acquiring the feeling that drinking is either prestigious, manly (and womanly) conduct, the equivalent of friendship and camaraderie, or the high road to the good life, virility, and all the other positive values.

In between the commercials, the entertainment content does nothing to dispute these claims; in fact, it reinforces them. It seems that cinema directors have settled on the idea that the only way to project strong emotions involving severe pressure or desperate decision making on the screen is to have the actor gulp drinks. A one-gulp scene appears to be equated to lesser pressures such as a rough day at work, but four or five gulps mean serious trouble. A recent television film showed the male lead downing shot after shot of what must have been strong tea because obvious signs of intoxication did not appear. This and a stern face were how he portrayed how desperate things were with him. Does such permeating propaganda cause or contribute to eventual alcoholism in some people?

Preoccupation with drink and securing one's supply lines are evidence of psychological dependence. The stash may be placed in the gastrointestinal tract in anticipation of an evening when potable beverages will not be provided. It may be in the car, on the person, or concealed around the house or garden, just in case the normal availability of alcohol is threatened, as on Election Day.

THE MANY ROADS TO ALCOHOLISM

There are many mental attitudes that help produce a problem drinker or an alcohol addict. The following list provides some of the proven approaches to achieving the status of being an alcoholic, and these should be considered danger signals.

• Ignore the need for morning drinks to control tremulousness as being anything of consequence.

• Pay no attention to the fact that you have blacked out during a drinking bout or two.

• Having had the DTs means that you were, by definition, addicted to alcohol. Not doing anything about it perpetuates the situation.

• Do not listen to anyone—family, friends, or doctors—who advises you to stop or markedly cut down on your drinking.

• If you do decide to stop or cut back and find you can't, well, you tried.

• If you have had a series of accidents while drunk, don't worry about it. You only drink as much as the other guys.

• If you find you're losing your ability to drink without getting drunk, it's not important.

• My father and grandfather were drunks so what's the use of fighting it?

• If it weren't for booze, you'd be a nervous wreck.

• There's nothing wrong with persistent thinking of the next drink, giving drinking high priority, and assuring that one's supplies are sufficient to take care of dry spells.

• You can't be an alcoholic. You only go on binges for a couple of weeks —two or three times a year.

SUMMARY

The drinking of the alcoholic differs in a number of ways from the drinking of a person who has no problems with the drug and who is not addicted to it. The wide diversity of alcoholic persons makes universal statements difficult, but certain behaviors that foster unsafe drinking are present with fair regularity in alcoholics.

The alcoholic seems to depend on alcohol as an exclusive technique of dealing with stress, boredom, and other unpleasant emotional states. Alcoholics have difficulty being realistic about their use of alcohol. The fact that they drank modestly for years and that the pattern has increased drastically is ignored or rationalized. Alcohol becomes a dominant and, eventually, an exclusive theme of existence. The stimulus-response aspect of drinking generalizes so that while, at one time, drinking was restricted to certain situations, eventually it becomes a response to all situations. Some of the difficulties of treating the alcoholic person arise from these differences.

22. The Myth of Controlled Drinking by Alcoholics

It was four years ago that an essay with the title: "Alcoholics: Can They Become Social Drinkers?" was published in *The Substance Abuse Problems*. It was written in response to an analysis of the first Rand report[1] which suggested that gamma alcoholics (addicted alcoholics) could be trained to become social drinkers. A number of flaws in the report were noted at that time and will not be mentioned here.

Since that time two important developments have taken place. One is the issuance of a second Rand report.[2] The second is an article by Pendery, Malzman, and West[3] seriously questioning the conclusions of the Sobell and Sobell[4,5] work. Since this investigation was the first controlled study that tested the controlled drinking hypothesis, it had considerable influence on the attitudes of many students of the subject.

THE SECOND RAND REPORT

The authors of the Rand report have explicitly stated, following the second study, that they "do not recommend that any alcoholic should resume drinking." When the original sample was restudied after a four-year period, the results of the first study were not confirmed. Those who had been drinking moderately at the six- and eighteen-month data collection periods tended to relapse. The second report seems to confirm a vast amount of clinical experience: Chronic alcoholics cannot drink small amounts of alcohol successfully over time.

THE SOBELL AND SOBELL PAPERS

In a study done at Patton State Hospital, California, during 1970–71, the Sobells compared 20 alcoholics who were trained to drink moderately by

128

behavioral methods with 20 who received conventional abstinence-oriented treatment. This was the seminal research test of the idea that physically dependent patients who had manifested loss of control over their drinking could be converted into social drinkers.

Method

The controlled drinking group received 17 individualized behavior therapy sessions in a simulated bar set up in the hospital. In the first two sessions up to 16 ounces of whiskey or its equivalent in other beverages were consumed, and the proceedings were videotaped. In the third session the patients sampled small amounts of a variety of mixed drinks to familiarize them with the diluted beverages and to demonstrate what social drinking behavior was like. The next 13 meetings were devoted to electric shock aversion-conditioning procedures interspersed with three no-shock sessions. Shocks were administered for such inappropriate behaviors as ordering straight drinks, not sipping the drinks, or ordering drinks too frequently.

The videotapes were played back to show the patients how they behaved while drunk. The patients were also trained in handling situations that had led to heavy drinking in the past. In the last session videotapes of their drunken and sober behaviors were compared, and the agreed-upon treatment goals reviewed. Upon completion of the program a card was given to each patient indicating that he or she was trained as a social drinker, with instructions about sipping mixed drinks, spacing drinks, and setting a moderate cutoff point for imbibing.

The Sobells reported that they followed each subject with contacts every three to four weeks and supplemented the interviews with official record reviews and other people's reports. Any discrepancies between these sources were extensively probed. They followed 19 of the 20 patients for two years after discharge. One patient was lost to them. One year later Caddy et al.[6] did an independent followup. Their report was likewise favorable to the idea that the controlled drinking subjects were performing very well.

Results

The unit of comparison between the experimental and control groups was the number of days each functioned well. After two years the controlled drinking group were significantly improved on this criterion at the .001 level for year two. The controlled drinking subjects also required far less incarceration or hospitalization according to the Sobells' observations. Overall, the controlled drinkers were described as having successfully achieved and sustained social drinking.

THE PENDERY, MALTZMAN, AND WEST ASSESSMENT
OF THE SOBELLS' WORK

Beginning five years after the Sobells' study, Pendery et al. restudied the controlled drinking subjects, their contacts, and their records of hospitalization, arrests, etc. The ability to find all 19 of the 20 subjects tracked by the Sobells is a testament to the diligence and thoroughness of the Pendery group.

Results

A very considerable discrepancy exists between the Sobells' papers and that of Pendery et al. Of the 16 subjects who originally fulfilled the criteria for gamma alcoholics, 13 had been rehospitalized within one year of completion of their social drinking training. Of these, 10 were returned to the Patton State Hospital alcoholism program, the same program where the Sobells were employed. The remaining 3 (of the 16) also abused alcohol over the three years following their treatment. The Sobells' comments on the need for rehospitalization of their controlled drinkers had suggested that they were voluntary admissions, "to curb the start of a binge, or to avoid drinking at all." Pendery and associates came to a vastly different interpretation. They found that the readmissions were caused by serious problem drinking or physical debility caused by alcohol.

The last 4 of the 20 controlled drinking subjects admitted to the study were not gamma, but alpha alcoholics (psychologically, not physically dependent). Three of these subjects also did poorly in subsequent years with intermittent excessive drinking, other drug usage, and multiple alcohol-related arrests. The fourth subject has been able to maintain his drinking at a moderate level to the present time. Thus, only 1 of the 20 controlled drinking subjects can be considered a successful social drinker, and he was an alpha alcoholic.

The fate of the 19 failures is enlightening. Six have stopped drinking completely after disastrous attempts to drink in a controlled manner. Four have died of alcohol-related causes. Eight continue to drink excessively, and all have experienced serious social and physical sequellae of alcohol excess. The one subject who could not be found had been certified as gravely disabled from drinking one year after completion of his behavioral treatment at Patton State Hospital.

THE ADDICTION RESEARCH FOUNDATION INQUIRY[7]

The Sobells are now employed at the Toronto-based Addiction Research Foundation. Following the Pendery et al. article in *Science*, a committee was formed to investigate the allegations made in that article. The committee concluded that, except for one lapse due to carelessness, and fewer than the stated number of follow-up interviews, the findings were accurately reported.

Unfortunately, the key issue was never examined by the committee: *Did the controlled drinking subjects control their drinking over time?* This is the vital question that is a life-or-death matter for the alcohol-dependent person who is placed on a social drinking program.

Is further research into controlled drinking for physically dependent alcoholics justified? It may not be, in view of the poor results of the two studies upon which this treatment goal is based. The abstinence-based programs have two obvious advantages. One, it removes the toxic product, and two, if any amount of alcohol is consumed, the danger signal is obvious. A social drinking alcoholic does not have this immediately evident signal to recognize impending relapse.

DISCUSSION

The significance of the Sobell and Sobell study is the influence it has had on many people involved in treatment and clinical research of alcoholism. A series of articles has been published during the past 10 years supporting or refuting their findings. A number of clinics and therapists now employ the goal of controlled drinking for their physically dependent patients. In view of the disappointing results of the second Rand report and the Pendery et al. review of the Sobells' research, it would be prudent to re-evaluate the controlled drinking treatment procedure. It is dangerous and rarely successful over the long term. In fact it may not be ethically justifiable to expose a gamma alcoholic to a controlled drinking goal.

The merits of behavior therapy are not at issue. It appears that for certain conditions, it may be successful. But its use in attempting to convert the gamma alcoholic to a social drinker is open to serious question.

One insufficiently discussed point in the controlled drinking controversy is that some chronic alcoholics may have such precarious liver, heart, brain, or pancreatic compensation that even the amount of alcohol consumed during successful controlled drinking may produce decompensation of one or more organs.

It may be that selected alpha alcoholics might justifiably have a single supervised trial of controlled drinking. But the question arises: Why take the risk? It is just as easy to be sociable with a soft drink in one's hand as with some mixed drink. If alcohol is being used as a means of stress management, the outlook over the long term is ominous for the psychologically dependent drinker. Among other options, behavioral therapy aimed at learning stress reduction techniques is preferred.

REFERENCES

1. Armor, J.D. et al. *Alcoholism and Treatment*. Rand Corp., 1700 Main St., Santa Monica, CA 90406, R1739-NIAAA, 1976.
2. Polich, J.M. The Course of Alcoholism: Four Years after Treatment. Rand Corp., Santa Monica, CA 90406, R2433-NIAAA, 1980.
3. Pendery, M.L. et al. Controlled drinking by alcoholics? New findings and a reevaluation of a major affirmative study. Science, 217:169-175, 1982.
4. Sobell, M.B. and Sobell, L.C. Behavior Therapy Research. 11:559, 1973.
5. Sobell, M.B. and Sobell, L.C. *Behavioral Treatment of Alcohol Problems*. Plenum, New York, 1978.
6. Caddy, G.R. et al. Behavior Therapy Research. 16:345, 1978.
7. Norman. C. No fraud found in alcoholism study. Science 218:771, 1982.

23. Alcohol and Malnutrition

Alcoholism may be the leading cause of malnutrition in the United States. For many reasons the usual recommended daily requirements of the various nutrients do not apply to the person ingesting large amounts of ethanol chronically. It is likely that every cell in the body is adversely affected by chronic alcoholism, but only certain organ systems are sufficiently impaired to become clinically obvious.

Ethanol provides 7.1 calories per gram (or about 200 calories an ounce). This means that a pint of 86 proof whiskey contains about 1,300 calories, about half the daily energy requirement for a sedentary person. Despite this caloric intake, the alcoholic may lose weight because of insufficient food intake and the gastrointestinal, hepatic, and pancreatic disorders that accompany alcoholism. Furthermore, calories from alcohol do not metabolize as well as carbohydrate. They do not form high energy phosphate bonds.

DIETARY DEFICIENCIES

The alcoholic's diet is usually inadequate either in all nutrients or in specific factors. The chronic drinker may be unwilling to spend money on food or may eat junk foods. A persistent loss of appetite for food may result from alcoholic gastritis, pancreatitis or hepatitis, or from ill-defined abdominal distress.

Malabsorption

The absorption of the water-soluble vitamins, notably folate, thiamine, and B12, is impaired during drinking. The assimilation of a number of nutrients across the small intestinal mucosa can be adversely affected. These include amino acids, glucose, water, electrolytes, and thiamine. Active drinking inhibits the secretion of pancreatic digestive enzymes. Folate and protein deple-

133

tion contribute to intestinal malabsorption including the absorption of folate itself.

Diarrhea and steatorrhea in the alcoholic are produced by intestinal hypermotility, pancreatic insufficiency inducing lipid malabsorption, cirrhosis, and intestinal flora changes. Not only are fat, water, and electrolytes lost, but also calcium, phosphate, zinc, and magnesium.

Disturbed Nutrient Metabolism

Ethanolism inhibits albumin synthesis resulting in albumin-globulin ratio reversal. Gluconeogenesis is disturbed and vitamin utilization is impaired. For example, the conversion of thiamine into its active form, thiamine pyrophosphate, the transformation of folic acid to its active component that is necessary for DNA synthesis, and the formation of pyridoxal phosphate from pyridoxine, are all disturbed. In addition, the damaged liver has poor storage capacity for most vitamins.

The metabolism of alcohol distorts lipid metabolism so that less is oxidized and more is converted to triglyceride. The excess of triglycerides appears as very low density lipoproteins in the serum with subsequent hyperlipidemia.

In addition to lowered intake, the fat-soluble vitamins are poorly absorbed in the small intestine when steatorrhea is present. This can lead to poor dark adaption and deficient spermatogenesis (vitamin A), or osteonecrosis and increased bone fractures (vitamin D and calcium). Vitamin K is also poorly absorbed and suffers from a decreased synthesis due to changes in the intestinal flora. Vitamin K lack can prolong prothrombin time and lead to clotting problems.

Increased Nutrient Requirements

The body's efforts at restitution of tissues destroyed by alcohol, the bleeding, and the infections to which the heavily drinking group is prone increase energy and vitamin requirements. Thiamin, riboflavin, folate, pyridoxine, and nicotinic acid all are involved in cellular repair processes and DNA and RNA synthesis.

Only a minority of alcoholics show an iron deficiency anemia. This is usually caused by substantial bleeding episodes. Wine, and to a lesser extent beer, contain iron so that intake is ordinarily adequate. What is more likely is an iron overload. Deficiencies of folate, B12, and particularly pyridoxine can disrupt the incorporation of iron into hemoglobin, producing an iron excess. When alcohol stimulates acid secretion in the stomach, it increases the absorption of ferric ions. These cannot be used for hemoglobin synthesis and are deposited in various tissues. Secondary hemochromatosis occurs in alcoholics. Supplementary iron and blood transfusions should only be given if a substantial iron deficiency anemia is present.

MALNUTRITION AND ORGAN DAMAGE

Functional and structural organ impairment caused by alcoholism results both from the toxic effects of alcohol or its metabolites and from the unavailability of essential nutrients.

Liver

High-protein diets have been shown to have a relative protective effect upon the liver during heavy drinking. However, even when an adequate balanced diet is consumed, large amounts of alcohol (more than 50 percent of the caloric intake) will cause fatty, inflammatory, and eventually scarifying changes.

Gastrointestinal Tract

Both alcohol and malnutrition contribute to the gastrointestinal and pancreatic damage in chronic alcoholics. Exocrine enzymatic deficiencies and anatomic alterations like erosive gastritis and jejunitis are seen. These latter are caused by disruption of the mucosal barrier by alcohol.

The synergistic action of alcohol and malnutrition is demonstrated by feeding a folate-deficient diet alone or providing alcohol alone. Each will cause no malabsorption of folic acid or xylose. Combining the two conditions results in folic acid and xylose malabsorption.

Cardiovascular System

The two kinds of alcoholic cardiomyopathy are beriberi heart due to thiamine deficiency and alcoholic (or perhaps acetaldehyde) cardiomyopathy caused by a direct toxic effect upon the heart muscle. Infrequently, they will occur together.

Hematopoietic and Immune Systems

Folate deficiency leads to megaloblastosis and megaloblastic anemia. Severe folate deficiencies can cause pancytopenia. Folate deficiency is evident when macrocytic erythrocytes are seen, or when an increased mean corpuscular volume (MCV) and a normal mean corpuscular hemoglobin (MCH) are reported on the complete blood count. This is rather common in the alcohol-dependent person.

Malnourished alcoholics have a lower percentage of circulating T lymphocytes, and they seem to have a reduced immune response capability. This is one of the reasons for an increased susceptibility to infection. Poor resistance to infection is also caused by a lifestyle without particular concern for proper hygiene, hypovitaminosis, and zinc deficiency.

Bleeding can result from gastritis, peptic ulceration, varices, the frequent traumas that accompany intoxication, low vitamin K levels, or thrombocytopenia due to alcohol, or folate insufficiency.

Nervous System

A number of vitamins, notably thiamine, nicotinic acid, pyridoxine, and B12, are essential for proper neuronal function. Although thiamine deficiency can be detected in a third of all alcoholics, less than 10 percent show evidence of the Wernicke-Korsakoff syndrome. Before the full-blown syndrome becomes evident, some patients will simply present symptoms of depression and mild memory and cognitive impairment. Nicotinic acid deficiency can cause pellagra with the dementia sometimes preceding the diarrhea and dermatitis.

The alcoholic peripheral neuropathy can have varying degrees of sensori-motor loss. If the earlier symptoms and signs are included, a third to a half of all alcoholics will be found with peripheral neuritis. Although it is ordinarily considered to be a thiamine lack complication, some patients do not recover until the entire B complex has been provided.

MANAGEMENT OF MALNOURISHED ALCOHOLICS

While the diagnosis, especially the early diagnosis of the various deficiencies that the malnourished alcoholic has, can be difficult, their treatment is relatively straightforward. Alcohol intake must cease. A well-balanced diet must be eaten or provided parenterally. Multivitamin therapy should be instituted. For those who want an objective confirmation of specific deficiencies, laboratory tests are available. The alcoholic's difficulties with absorption and their conversion to active forms make large doses of the essential vitamins rational. During the early phase of treatment injectable administration may be required. Chronic infections including dental caries and abcesses should receive treatment. If intravenous glucose is given to a seriously vitamin-deficient patient, an acute avitaminosis may be precipitated. Parenteral water-soluble vitamins should be provided.

In addition to the usual cautions regarding large doses of vitamin A and routine administration of iron, care should be exercised with protein supplementation. Liver failure may restrict the patient's ability to deal with even ordinary amounts of protein without inducing an encephalopathy due to ammonia accumulation.

SUMMARY

The nutritional deficiencies of the alcoholic may be multiple and severe. Malnutrition compounds the toxic effects of alcohol. Early diagnosis of the nutrient inadequacies may avoid future organ damage.

BIBLIOGRAPHY

- Karsten, M.A. and Lieber, C.S. Nutrition and the alcoholic. Med. Clinics North Amer. 63: 963-972, 1979.
- Morgan, M.Y. Alcohol and nutrition: In: *Alcohol and Disease*. Ed.: S. Sherlock, New York, Churchill-Livingstone, 1982.
- Schmitz, R.E. Nutritional assessment in the alcoholic. Advances in Alcoholism. 2: (2), 1981.
- Shaw, S. and Lieber, C.S. Nutrition and Alcoholism. In: *Modern Nutrition in Health and Disease,* 6th Ed. Eds.: R.S. Goodhart and M.E. Shils, Philadelphia, Lea and Febiger, 1979.

24. Alcohol and the American Indian

Very few American Indian tribes had contact with alcohol in any form, and none had knowledge of distilled spirits until the early contacts with European settlers. Beer and wine were used in a few areas, but only in connection with religious ceremonies. As the frontier expanded during the eighteenth century, traders soon discovered that providing "firewater" to the Indian lubricated the bartering process. Negotiating trade or treaty agreements with intoxicated Indians was a common exploitative process.

It is believed that Indians adopted their drinking practices from the frontiersman and later the cowboy who tended to drink rapidly till drunk and then exhibit unrestrained or violent behavior. Although many generations have passed since the frontier vanished, it is possible that these role models still influence current consumption styles.

In addition, the intoxicated state may have meshed with the cultural matrix of certain tribal groups. For example, an important component of the Iroquois' traditional spiritual exercises was the achievement of an ecstatic experience. It has been suggested that some of their drive to drink to intoxication and beyond represented a search to achieve an "out-of-body" state. The Sioux sun dance was also a strenuous effort to disassociate, and the "sacred water" might represent an inferior attempt to fill the void of deculturation and a quest for visionary experience.

Whether it was for reasons such as these, or because of the loss of self-respect, homelands, or the ancient spiritual solidarity, the Amerindian population has long had problems with alcohol. In an effort to deal with a deteriorating situation, Indian leaders requested a law forbidding the sale of alcoholic beverages to Indians. In 1832 Congress passed such legislation. This early effort at prohibition did not remedy the situation. Bootlegging and other evasive practices quickly arose. It compelled the buyer to rapidly and completely consume the whiskey. Indians never had the opportunity to learn how to drink moderately or to develop social taboos against drunken comportment.

In 1953, this discriminating and ineffective law was repealed and prohibition became a tribal option. It is interesting to note that 70 percent of the reservations have retained the prohibition on reservation property. Its value is open to question.

EXTENT OF THE PROBLEM

The statistics are grim and the trend shows no evidence of improvement. Alcoholism among Indians is more than two and maybe as much as four times the national level and is higher than for any other minority group. Accidental deaths are first among the causes of death for native Americans, accounting for a fifth of all deaths. The Indian Health Service estimates that 75 percent of the injuries and deaths are alcohol related.

The first ten causes of death among Indians show five that are directly or indirectly due to alcohol overuse. These account for 35 percent of Indian mortality, shortening the life span significantly and causing enormous morbidity. They are:

- Accidents   21 percent
  (75 percent alcohol related)

- Cirrhosis   6 percent
  (compared with 1.7 percent nationally)

- Alcoholism   3.2 percent
  (four times the national average)

- Suicide   2.9 percent
  (twice the national average)
  (80 percent alcohol related)

- Homicide   2 percent
  (90 percent alcohol related)

In addition, alcoholic pancreatitis, heart disease, malnutrition, and peptic ulceration contribute to the number of fatalities sometimes associated with heavy drinking.

Male Indians drink more and have more problems related to drinking, but the female Indian drinking rate is also at a high level. In fact, it equals the male Anglo rate. The incidence of fetal alcohol syndrome seems to be disproportionately high among newborn Indian infants, but additional studies must be done to confirm this.

ETIOLOGIC ASPECTS

It has long been claimed that Indians metabolize alcohol less effectively than Caucasians; therefore they are more prone to develop the social and physiologic complications of drinking. This means that less would affect them more. A number of studies have been done with variable results. It appears that other factors are more important in explaining the physiological and behavioral toxicity.

Since the American Indian is of Mongolian ancestry, it can be assumed that some will have the Oriental flush syndrome. This condition does occur with some frequency in the Indian population. In one study 50 percent of Cree Indians flushed after a small test dose. The flush is presumed to be caused by high acetaldehyde levels, perhaps because of deficient aldehyde dehydrogenase activity. Since the flush itself is experienced as unpleasant, and in severe cases, is accompanied with asthma and tachycardia, it should be somewhat of a deterrent to alcohol consumption. Although, in a few instances, this may be true, it certainly is not a group-protective metabolic aberration. Needless to say, it does not explain the Indians' problem with ethanol.

Cultural, social, and familial factors are more important than biochemical or metabolic alterations. The contribution of idiosyncratic cultural forms to overdrinking is impressive when considering various tribal alcoholism prevalence rates. The Cherokee alcohol-related death rate is only 6/100,000. Among the Cheyenne-Arapahos it is 239/100,000.

It must not be assumed that Indian drinking patterns are monolithic or uniform. They vary markedly from tribe to tribe. Sixty percent of Navahos are complete abstainers from alcohol. This compares with about 25 percent in the general population. Some of the Plains Indian groups tend to be most involved with dysfunctional drinking practices.

Urban and rural Indians show different patterns of use. The former group consumes less alcohol and displays drinking styles that tend to conform as much to their social class as to their tribal origin. Middle-class Indians in a large city drink more like middle-class Anglos than like poorer Indians. It is probable that the social factors that alienate people, like unemployment, discrimination, and transitional acculturation, play a role in excessive drinking behaviors. Those who have neither roots in their traditional Indian heritage nor a stake in the dominant society are at the greatest risk. Among rural Indian alcoholics, boredom, hopelessness, and the periodic need to release suppressed feeling must contribute to the binge-type drinking observed there.

PATTERNS OF DRINKING

What will be described are drinking patterns that are more characteristic of Indians than of other groups. It should not be viewed as a stereotype, since Indians, like all populations, present a wide variety of drinking customs.

Drinking is often an extended kin group-oriented activity. Communal imbibing is considered a sign of friendship and cohesiveness. Group drinking, sometimes in the form of "passing the bottle," is a norm. Collections are taken to purchase the beverage and noncontributors are expected to "party." In fact, the strong pressures exerted by the group to drink along contribute to the relapse rate of those who are attempting to remain abstinent. Refusing a drink is tantamount to insulting the offerer. Solitary drinking is infrequent.

Drinking starts early in life and may be preceded by gasoline or other solvent sniffing. There is little interference with an individual's drinking or drunken comportment. The point of consuming is to get drunk, so the beverage is ingested rapidly until it is gone or until the user is stuporous. This sort of blitz drinking leads to quick intoxication. Little attempt is made to conceal one's drunkenness; actually, it may occasionally be exaggerated. "Raising hell" is common: loud, boisterous acting out, accompanied by manifest aggressive and sexual conduct. Despite the apparent loss of controls, efforts not to "mess up" are discernible. When enforcement officials are present, imbibers will "cool it." That this is not too successful is indicated by the finding that 76 percent of all adult Native Americans' arrests are alcohol related. One member of the group may remain sober so that he or she can drive the others from bar to bar. Nevertheless, the conviction rate for Native Americans driving while intoxicated was seven times greater than the proportion of Indian drivers in the total driving population. Such "cruising" is commonly practiced in urban situations, especially on weekends. Indian bars are prime meeting and socializing places. They tend to be animated and loud, and the patrons socialize more than in equivalent Anglo bars.

This binge type of fast alcohol ingestion overwhelms the body's mechanisms for dealing with ethanol. Very high blood alcohol levels must be reached quickly, providing little opportunity for the user to adapt to the profound psychophysiological effects. Death from alcohol overdose is known to occur under such circumstances, but a more frequent concern is the complete loss of control over behavior.

PREVENTION AND TREATMENT

An important requirement would be an entirely new attitude toward alcohol by the Indian youth. At present, the policy of placing few family and social sanctions on the young person's drinking, the excessive drinking role models provided by older relatives, and the symbolic rewards from drunkenness all contribute to perpetuate destructive drinking practices. An entire generation of children will have to be educated about the self-destructive and genocidal nature of current alcohol consuming styles and provided with alternative forms of socializing and enjoying. Otherwise, the process continues and a third of the Indian population succumbs to the multiple lethalities of this single drug.

The bulk of the treatment services offered by the Indian Health Service is oriented toward problem drinking and its antisocial and physiological sequelae. Many of these are conventional: detoxification, counselling, AA, or hospital care for trauma or medical disorders. Treatment methods have to be integrated into the distinctive Indian tradition and community support obtained; otherwise, intervention is destined to fail.

Detoxification and urban alcohol recovery centers are no more successful than their Anglo counterparts, even when staffed with Indian exalcoholics. When they are located in the skid rows of metropolitan areas, they are perceived not as opportunities to recover, but as a chance to obtain the food, medical care, and services needed to rehabilitate enough to venture out on another bout. Another advantage to the consumer is that the time spent in a recovery home produces a decrease in tolerance so that less alcohol will have a greater mind-altering effect.

The traditional AA group conflicts with the Indian tradition of not discussing personal problems and confessing in public. A few AA-oriented Indian lodges have employed the stratagem of having alcoholics regale the group with a lively description of their prowess ih defeating the enemy, the bottle, just as their forefathers related the dangers and triumphs of the battle and hunting trips.

Treatment methods indigenous to the culture also exist. Some medicine men attempt to instill pride in the tribal heritage as a basis for change toward sobriety. Some are using the root of the trumpet vine as an Antabuse-like deterrent. It is said to make the effects of alcohol less pleasant.

One of the more interesting approaches to the management of the alcoholic is practiced by the Native American church. One of the tenets of the church is sobriety, but when someone slips, the peyote ceremony is used as a treatment. The ritual use of the peyote cactus utilizing traditional rituals is believed to have lead to sobriety for some members, although statistics hardly exist. What the peyote ceremony contributes is a depersonalized state of great hypersuggestibility, which, when guided by the Road Man, provides an experience of self-transcendence and communion with the Great Spirit. Personal problems are not examined. Instead, the supplicant's destructive lifestyle is clearly seen, either symbolically or in actual vivid pictures. The Right Way is indicated, and if things go well, the alcoholic reforms his or her life into a more constructive style.

Intoxication has been suggested by some anthropologists, and no less a psychologist than William James, as being an effort to achieve a higher spiritual consciousness, a state which is highly valued in many Indian cultures. If so, alcohol intoxication is a poor one for this purpose. Peyote provides a much more dramatic, palpable, impressive theobotanical experience. It is unfortunate that the long-term results of peyote exposure cannot be reliably determined insofar as alcohol abstinence is concerned.

BIBLIOGRAPHY

- Albough, B.J. and Anderson, P. Peyote in the treatment of alcoholism among American Indians. Am. J. Psychiat. 131:1247-1257, 1974.
- Alcohol and Health. Third Special Report to the Congress, U.S. Government Printing Office, Washington, D.C. 1978.
- Alcohol and Health. Fourth Special Report to the Congress, U.S. Government Printing Office, Washington, D.C. 1981.
- Burns, M. et al. Drinking practices and problems of urban American Indians in Los Angeles. Planning Analysis and Research Institute, Santa Monica, CA 1974.

25. The Aging
Social Drinker

This essay is not about geriatric alcoholism. It deals with the effects of small amounts of alcohol upon the process of aging with emphasis upon mental functioning. What is true for most psychoactive drugs is valid for alcohol: small amounts are likely to have opposite effects than large quantities have. Small amounts are arbitrarily defined here as no more than two average-sized drinks once or twice a day. Aging is, of course, a lifelong process, but for purposes of this discussion, it is arbitrarily considered to be the period after age 60.

THE AGING PROCESS

The general impression is, after excluding the group with dementia of the Alzheimer type, that the "normally" aging person sustains a gradual, linear, cognitive impairment over the years. The research on this point is variable. Jarvik mentions "from our own research at the New York State Psychiatric Institute, if illness does not intervene, cognitive stability is the rule and can be maintained into the ninth decade." Eisdorfer has found that intellectual decline correlates better with an elevated diastolic blood pressure than with age, at least until the eighth decade. Many authors have shown, on the other hand, that aging is accompanied by a number of performance and cognitive deficits. Wechsler, in fact, stated that most human abilities decline progressively after the mid-20s. This position has been questioned by subsequent research.

Many of these conclusions apparently depend on what cognitive functions are being studied. Those tests which measure elements of crystallized intelligence (accumulated knowledge) improve at least into the 60s, while those that measure new learning and problem solving (fluid intelligence) tend to drop off. The same process seems to be valid for memory. Long-term memorial stores and recognition memory are much less affected by age than the retrieval of recently acquired memories.

144

Thus, while the healthy, aging population retains a fair cognitive ability, a gradual decrement in certain functions is undeniable. A proper question that can be asked is: Is the cognitive functional loss during the sober interval accentuated by alcohol in amounts that are not presumed to produce mental impairment in the younger age groups?

THE WERNICKE-KORSAKOFF SYNDROME

Chronic brain damage caused by alcohol is second only to Alzheimer's syndrome in frequency among adult populations. Some of the symptoms of the two mental conditions are similar: for example, the loss of ability to think abstractly, speech difficulties, and decreased coordination. Other manifestations, like polyneuritis and occulomotor paralyses, differentiate the two conditions. Patients from both groups show brain-wave abnormalities and, eventually, cerebral atrophy. Alzheimer's encephalopathy seems to be more progressive, but alcoholic deterioration may be arrested or even improved with abstinence and proper nutrition. The similarity of the two conditions makes the question about the aging person being more vulnerable to the psychological effects of alcohol a reasonable inquiry.

SOME BENEFITS OF SOCIAL DRINKING UPON AGING

1. One or two drinks a day lowers the blood pressure a few millimeters. Large amounts of ethyl alcohol will increase blood pressure, and it may remain high during sober intervals.

2. Survival rates of consumers of small amounts of alcohol are slightly better than of abstainers insofar as death from coronary artery disease is concerned. Alcoholics, though, have a higher mortality from heart attacks than nonusers or social users.

3. In studies of individuals in senior citizen homes, it has usually been found that a beer or a glass of light wine improves sociability and mood and decreases negative attitudes toward patients and staff. This is particularly true when the beverage is served in a pub setting.

4. In social situations small amounts of alcohol seem to reduce tension, lift mood, and relax social interactions. These changes are opposite in direction to the impact of heavy drinking upon mood, especially in the aged.

5. A general cultural belief exists that certain alcoholic drinks (aperitifs) increase the appetite. Alcohol is known to increase gastric acid secretion, and

perhaps it improves appetite on that basis. This has apparently not been critically tested, but if true, would be helpful in old people with anorexia.

SOME ADVERSE CONSEQUENCES
OF SOCIAL DRINKING UPON AGING

1. Alcohol is the ultimate junk food. It contains empty calories, and certain vitamins are expended in its metabolism. Elderly social drinkers who may obtain about 400 calories a day from their alcohol-containing beverages could develop a shortage of the vitamin B complex, especially if their diet happens to be marginal in its vitamin content.

2. Even small amounts of ethanol cannot be recommended for people with certain illnesses like liver disease, moderate or severe diabetes, or peptic ulcers. Individuals with these conditions should be abstainers. Those who require drugs with tranquilizing or sedating actions may find that combining such drugs with small amounts of alcohol increases drowsiness and decreases driving ability.

3. Some elderly people will find that their previous ability to drink even social amounts of fermented or distilled beverages is impaired, and that one drink produces dizziness or some impairment of mentation. This sensitivity may be related to a loss of one's previous control over the psychological effects of alcohol due to neuronal degenerative changes. It should also be recalled that aging brings with it a reduced volume of distribution resulting from a reduced body water and lean body mass in old people. These alterations will increase the blood and brain alcohol concentration.

THE EFFECT OF SOCIAL DRINKING ON
COGNITION IN THE AGING

Several research investigations have found that those who consume more than five drinks a day display a poorer cognitive performance while sober than their light-drinking or nondrinking counterparts. Other studies have determined that age was a strong risk factor in the decline in abstraction ability among sober heavy drinkers. It was natural to inquire into the influence of social drinking on an aging population.

Parker et al. completed two investigations utilizing middle-aged and elderly adults who drank five or fewer drinks a day. The subjects were asked about their alcohol consumption in the past. Detailed information was obtained about their drinking patterns during the past month, in particular about the quantity and frequency of each drinking episode.

A standard test of vocabulary and abstraction (the Shipley Institute of Living Scale) was administered during a nondrinking period. The rationale of the test is that in certain states of cognitive functioning, crystallized knowledge like vocabulary is less affected, but the ability to form new abstract relationships will be more disturbed in the aged. An average vocabulary score and a lowered abstraction score would point to difficulty in fluid intelligence like concept formation.

A number of recent studies of social drinkers have found that abstraction performance while sober decreases according to their drinking practices. Among a group of employed men and women, a significant relationship between the *quantity of alcohol consumed per drinking occasion* and their ability to abstract was found. The *frequency* of drinking was not significantly related to cognitive functioning. Whether a person had drunk alcohol within the past 24 hours was also of no consequence.

Lifetime consumption also failed to significantly predict cognitive impairment so long as quantity consumed on each drinking occasion remained low.

There was a linear relationship between the amount consumed per occasion and the abstraction deficit. Age also was shown to be a significant risk factor, with older age groups doing more poorly than younger groups.

Verbal intelligence remained fairly intact, but abstracting ability decreased. The total quantity of alcohol used was not as significant as the amount used on a typical drinking occasion. Apparently, it is the episodic concentration of alcohol (or acetaldehyde?) in the brain that produces the damage. This is an important point for the aging person. The ingestion of one or two drinks at a time on one or two occasions is less impairing of higher mental functions than if four or five units are drunk on a single occasion.

DISCUSSION

The conceptual changes that occur in aging people are subtle and not readily identifiable subjectively. When optimal mental performance is required, the inability to think abstractly may sometimes be noted by oneself or others. Abstinence does not seem to be required to avoid the cognitive slippage described. It is avoided by spacing drinks and eating while drinking, measures that keep brain alcohol concentrations low.

The aging individual who has sustained a partial loss of abstracting ability because of alcohol intake can recover some or all of the decrement. The alcohol-related decrement is reversible, and re-examination of such a person months or years following testing will show restoration of cognitive performance if abstinence or drinking of minimal amounts of alcoholic beverage has occurred in the interim.

The relationship between drinking too much episodically and subsequent sober performance cannot be considered causal. It is, at this point, merely a relationship. It may be that people with reduced cognitive performance drink more heavily when they drink, thereby accounting for the findings.

It must be emphasized that we are considering social drinking patterns. The story with alcoholics is quite different. Alcoholic men in their 40s have approximately the same memorial and perceptual abilities as nonalcoholic men in their late 50s. This functional aging of the central nervous system of alcoholics has been remarked upon by many clinicians and researchers. They agree, though, that part or all of the deficit is reversible provided complete abstinence is maintained over time.

The above information about the fact that even lower levels of drinking could be harmful to certain aspects of mental functioning is worth bringing to the attention of the aging social drinker. For those who prefer abstinence, this attitude can be supported. Those who prefer to drink moderately should be aware that consuming more than one or two average-sized drinks on a single occasion may produce undesired abstraction difficulties that can extend into the sober interval.

SUMMARY

Drinking habits change during the latter period of life. As a rule, less alcohol is consumed, intoxication is rare or nonexistent, and if binges were ever indulged in, they disappear. Of course, late-onset alcoholism can also emerge, but it is infrequent.

The diminished pattern of consumption may result from a perceived increased sensitivity. Whatever the reason, it is prudent that it occur at a time when the aging brain is becoming vulnerable to damage from more than modest amounts of the drug. An accelerated abstracting disability is likely when alcohol even in less than intoxicating amounts is imbibed by the elderly.

IV
OTHER MIND-ALTERING SUBSTANCES

26. Methaqualone: A New Twist

Methaqualone (Quaalude, Mecquin) has recently been withdrawn from the marketplace. However, some very new developments make it worthwhile to take another look at this troublesome sleeping pill. It was approved for prescription use in 1965 and placed in Schedule V, the least restrictive of all schedules, one that permitted unlimited refills. This turned out to be a costly miscalculation because it immediately became briskly abused. It had been sold as Mandrax in Great Britain and elsewhere prior to its introduction in the United States, and it had a history of abuse in a number of countries.

Methaqualone is the only drug that was upscheduled in one move from V to II, the latter being the most restrictive schedule for prescription drugs. Many states required the use of triplicate prescription forms for the drug.

THE MISUSE OF THE STRESS CLINIC CONCEPT

In recent years stress management clinics have emerged, perhaps in response to at least two developments. More people are seeking assistance in handling their stressful life situations. While this age is probably no more stress-engendering than most others, many individuals are unwilling to accept the burden of enduring tension and anxiety. In earlier times it was more customary to "tough out" psychological distress.

The second development is the emergence of helpful stress reduction techniques. These include biofeedback, self-hypnosis, meditation, relaxation exercises, and other interventions. The management program often includes behavior therapy in which the individual is trained to deal effectively with the specific stressful situations in his or her life. Alternatively, if the stresses can not be neutralized, then environmental adjustments are recommended. In general, antianxiety drugs do not constitute an important element of the treatment. Some stress clinics do not use them, others will prescribe them in combination with nondrug measures.

151

What is new and different at this time is the emergence of a number of "stress clinics" in major metropolitan areas that treat stress almost exclusively by prescribing 30 to 60 300 mg Quaalude tablets at a time, all the while capitalizing on the success of legitimate stress clinics. In an attempt to comply with the requirement that complete histories and physicals be performed before prescribing controlled drugs, the clinics employ some of the same self-rating life stress forms that are seen in the conventional stress management centers. The patient's responses do not seem to matter because in some cases, in less than five minutes an untrained "counselor" has approved the patient for Quaalude. It has been suggested that in some so-called stress clinics this brief interview is actually done to screen out nosy reporters and undercover state medical regulatory inspectors.

Who are the patients? They tend to be white, middle-class, young adults who appear at the clinic expressly for "ludes." Some of the self-rating forms that I have reviewed showed exposure to no more than the ordinary life stresses. These individuals apparently had not received instructions on how to fill out the form so that some justification for providing Quaalude might exist.

The only approved use of Quaalude is for the treatment of insomnia. No literature could be found that indicates that it has effectiveness as an antistress drug. It is evident on reviewing the charts, that many methaqualone "stress clinics" exist solely as a quasi-legal operation for the distribution of Quaaludes to those who want them. As indicated, the forms that are filled out in order to obtain a stress profile are less than perfunctory. The doctor's physical examination can hardly be revealing when known to consume as much as five minutes, but is usually briefer.

The economics involved are impressive. For the 10 minutes or so of staff time, a fee of $100.00 may be obtained. In some operations, the pharmacist may be linked to the operation financially, charging about $1.50 for each tablet, well in excess of the usual cost of Quaalude from nonclinic pharmacists. This means that the total cost to the patient is about $5.00 per tablet. The cost can be compared with the current price for a tablet sold illegally on the street, which is $10.00. A good profit can be made by the patient inclined to resell his or her supply.

The physicians involved may be recruited through the local newspaper's want ads. They may work only four to eight hours a week, and may clear $100.00 an hour or more. The reason why such brief tours of duty are arranged is to spread the large volume of Quaalude prescriptions among several different doctors so that it will not be apparent to the state monitors of controlled drugs that a prescription-mill operation exists.

It has been estimated that between 80 to 90 percent of all prescriptions for Quaalude in New York State last year originated in one "stress clinic." Half of all these prescriptions were allegedly filled in a single pharmacy.

Nonprofessional entrepreneurs usually own the clinics. It may be that a number of the clinics are owned by one person or a single syndicate. Quaalude-prescribing establishments have been closed down in New Jersey, Nevada, and Los Angeles. At the moment it is believed clinics in New York, Phoenix, Atlanta, Chicago, and a few in Miami are still open and functioning using available sedatives.

EPIDEMIOLOGY AND PHARMACOLOGY

In 1980, 5,300 emergency room "mentions" of methaqualone were recorded in the Drug Abuse Warning Network system, an increase of 137 percent in three years. This increase is due only in part to Quaalude clinic activity. A considerable number of methaqualone tablets, some made to look like Quaaludes, are manufactured outside the country and smuggled in. Three and a half tons of the substance are legitimately produced, and an estimated 100 tons cross the national boundary illegally. The reasons for the emergency room visits included side effects, interactions with other drugs, overdose, and withdrawal symptoms.

Side Effects

In therapeutic doses dry mouth, nausea, and mild dizziness might be noted. A hangover after awakening is a possibility. With larger than average amounts, cerebellar signs consisting of nystagmus, ataxia, and slurred speech can occur. Paradoxical excitement and restlessness are known to happen infrequently. Some patients complain of paresthesias, and a few instances of peripheral neuropathy have been reported. It is interesting that one other hypnotic, thalidomide, also causes peripheral neuropathies. Methaqualone has induced skeletal deformities in newborn rats, therefore the drug should not be used during pregnancy.

Interaction with Other Drugs

Naturally, combining methaqualone with other sedative-hypnotics and tranquilizers will have, at least, an additive effect. Mandrax is a methaqualone-diphenhydramine (Benadryl) mixture. Whether the Benadryl does more than add to the sedative activity is unknown. Since methaqualone is hydroxylated by the liver microsomal enzymes, its action is potentiated by alcohol, which utilizes the same metabolic system. The alcohol-methaqualone potentiation is well known on the street where it is deliberately produced and called "luding out."

Overdose

At prelethal levels severe myoclonus can develop, and it may require neuromuscular blockers for relief. The gag reflex might remain intact, making intubation difficult. The picture resembles barbiturate overdose with hypotension, apnea, stupor or restlessness, and delirium. Coma after 2.4 gm and death after 8.0 gm are known. On the other hand a survival following the ingestion of 22.0 gm is recorded. At death, blood levels of 0.5 to 2.5 mg/100 ml are usually found. If recovery occurs, amnesia for the episode is present.

Abstinence Syndrome

Tolerance will be clinically noted over a few weeks of taking two 300 mg tablets daily. At higher dosage levels tolerance will occur sooner. Suddenly discontinuing the daily use of four or more tablets can induce a sedative-type withdrawal syndrome. This includes tremulousness, insomnia, delirium, agitation, and late-onset major convulsions.

WHY IS QUAALUDE ABUSED?

It was originally believed that Quaalude was just one more hypnotic drug, and that its attractiveness was due to the intoxication and the relief from dysphoria that all drugs in this class provided. When Quaalude abusers called it "heroin for lovers" it was presumed that, like the barbiturates and alcohol, it led to increased desire as a consequence of its disinhibiting effect. It was assumed that the occasional allegations of improved erectile ability in males were also a reflection of diminished shyness, guilt, or overconcern about performing adequately. Thus the drug's ability to reduce sexual inhibitions was supposed to be due to a nonspecific sedative property. This question remains unsettled, and any sexual component of Quaalude's activity is incompletely understood. A small primate study indicates a possible aphrodisiac effect. Whether a specific aphrodisiac action is present is not known. Why the need exists for an aphrodisiac in the age groups that abuse Quaalude, is unclear.

Similarly, the need for young adults to take anti-insomnia medication unless severe pain or distress is present, is questionable. It would seem preferable to treat the primary cause of the insomnia. When hypnotics are needed, very short courses are almost invariably sufficient. The continued use of sleep medication is unwarranted, in fact, it is contraindicated. Therefore, the "stress clinics'" practice cannot be justified, and only harm can result. They actually represent an effort to supply a demand for Quaalude; it is drug dealing under a medical pretext.

Most Quaalude abuse is apparently for its sedative, nonsexual action. It would be worth knowing whether the subjective effects can be differentiated from barbiturates or benzodiazepines when administered to experienced users on a blind basis. It may be that much of the methaqualone popularity and the claims for it are based upon folklore.

WHAT CAN BE DONE?

Two issues are involved in the Quaalude question: one is the medical ethics of the so-called "stress clinics," and the second is the overall problem of methaqualone abuse.

These so-called "stress clinics" have no justification for their existence. They do not help people deal with stress; rather they compound their patients' problems by supporting or adding methaqualone dependence. It should be of particular concern to the medical profession that some of its members are knowingly involved in such operations.

Methaqualone's sleep-promoting ability can be duplicated or bettered by many other hypnosedatives. In view of its expanding nonmedical use the move has been made to delete the drug from the list of approved prescription drugs. Such a measure will not solve the overall problems with Quaalude, but it should be studied to determine its impact. Nevertheless, the total annual legal production is 3.5 tons, and that amount is estimated to be about 4 percent of the illicitly introduced material.

The abuse of methaqualone goes beyond the "stress clinic" matter. Supply reduction should be vigorously attempted. Most of the supplies come in from clandestine laboratories situated abroad. As part of the entire supply reduction program, methaqualone trafficking is best brought under control at the level of the manufacturing laboratory, or while being shipped in bulk across the border. Meanwhile, educational efforts and other prevention techniques are needed to reduce the demand.

27. The Anxiolytic Agents

The benzodiazepines constitute the primary group of drugs for the control of anxiety. They clearly are more effective and safer than other antianxiety agents such as phenobarbital and meprobamate. But the benzodiazepines are not only satisfactory for the treatment of anxiety and derivative conditions. They also have anticonvulsant, muscle relaxant, and hypnotic capabilities.

We will present recent benzodiazepine research findings, some guidelines for their rational use, and will provide a clinical differentiation between the two major subgroups of the benzodiazepines. A dozen benzodiazepines have been approved for marketing in the United States. Additional ones, quazepam, for example, are in various phases of the approval process.

Table 27–1[1] separates benzodiazepines according to their half-lives because short and long half-lives may be clinically significant. This is not to say that a short half-life is synonymous with a short duration of action. While certain benzodiazepines have been marketed for specific indications, it is likely that the entire class participates, to a greater or lesser degree, in all the therapeutic effects.

PHARMACOLOGY

The benzodiazepines are lipid soluble assuring gastrointestinal absorption within a half hour. Peak blood levels are found 60 to 90 minutes after oral ingestion. Plasma albumin binding (80 to 98 percent), active metabolites, and redistribution to fat stores account for the extended half-lives. The major metabolite for many of the long half-life drugs is nordesmethyldiazepam. Hydroxylation and glucuronide configuration is a frequent metabolic pathway.

The benzodiazepines are much safer than the barbiturates and are preferred for patients with some measure of suicidal inclinations. Two hundred to a thousand times the therapeutic dose has been deliberately consumed with subsequent recovery. More than a hundred times the average dose has been swallowed without inducing a deep coma.[2]

The presence of at least two specific benzodiazepine receptors has been

156

Table 27–1
Marketed Benzodiazepines

Generic Name	Trade Name	Special Indication
Short Half-Life (4 to 20 hours)		
Oxazepam	Serax	
Lorazepam	Ativan	
Temazepam	Restoril	Hypnotic
Alprazolam	Xanax	
Triazolam	Halcion	Hypnotic
Long Half-Life (24 to 72 hous)		
Chlordiazepoxide	Librium	
Diazepam	Valium	Status epilepticus
Chlorazepate	Tranxene, Azene	
Flurazepam	Dalmane	Hypnotic
Clonazepam	Clonopin	Petit mal
Prazepam	Verstran, Centrax	
Halazepam	Paxipam	

confirmed.[3] Type I is postulated to exert antianxiety activity and Type II is assumed to account for the sedative effect. The clinical finding that tolerance to sedation occurs before tolerance to the antianxiety effect is consistent with the dual receptor concept. The benzodiazepine receptors are situated in close relationship to gamma aminobutyric acid (GABA) receptors which are inhibitors of neural transmission. It is probable that benzodiazepines are GABA co-transmitters, dampening brain excitation. After extensive benzodiazepine therapy, GABA activity is reduced. Abrupt benzodiazepine discontinuance produces a rebound hyperactivity presumably because of low levels of GABA production.[3]

SHORT AND LONG HALF-LIFE BENZODIAZEPINES: COMMON PROPERTIES

Benzodiazepines are well absorbed because of their lipid solubility. Cross tolerance to other CNS depressants, like alcohol and barbiturates, exists. An additive effect should be anticipated when such combinations are taken. Physical dependence to all benzodiazepines can be observed at high doses or at average amounts when they are used for prolonged periods.

SHORT HALF-LIFE BENZODIAZEPINE: SPECIAL FEATURES

1. Cumulation can develop, but it is at a lower level than with the long half-life group.

2. The withdrawal syndrome comes on sooner. It is briefer, but more intense than the long half-life group. Myoclonus, insomnia, and nightmares are described. Seizures might occur one to four days after discontinuing the drug. Hollister[4] has collected 48 cases of postwithdrawal convulsions after stopping short half-life drugs, and additional reports have appeared since his report.

3. These drugs may be preferred for brief anxiety attacks.

4. When used as hypnotics they seem to produce more rebound insomnia[5] and early awakening.[6]

5. In cirrhotic or elderly patients they are more promptly excreted and may be preferable.

6. When used as an amnesic agent, intravenous lorazepam will take longer to pass the blood brain barrier but will also take longer to pass out of the barrier than will diazepam. Therefore, it is preferred when prolonged amnesia is desired as for cancer chemotherapy patients whose nausea and vomiting cannot be controlled.

LONG HALF-LIFE BENZODIAZEPINE: SPECIAL FEATURES

1. Fewer daily doses will be required for full-day coverage. Missing a dose is less likely to evoke emergent anxiety.

2. The withdrawal syndrome on sudden discontinuance is delayed. It will last longer, be less intense, and will taper off in a week or longer. Seizures may occur three to ten days after stopping the drug. The analogy that the short half-life benzodiazepines may be secobarbital-like in their withdrawal syndromes and the long half-life ones are phenobarbital-like may be appropriate.

3. This group is usually selected for extended anxiety attacks or when their onset is unpredictable.

4. These drugs cumulate for four to seven days, then achieve a steady state with elevated blood levels, but usually without sedation.

5. Intramuscular absorption of chlordiazepoxide and diazepam is delayed; therefore they should be used orally or intravenously.

6. Diazepam produces a brief amnesic period when given intravenously and is satisfactory for endoscopic procedures.

7. Chlorazepate and prazepam are pro-drugs. They are inactive, requiring gastric acid for conversion to active compounds. They should not be used in patients with anacidity or in those who take antacids frequently.

INDICATIONS

The benzodiazepines should not be used for mild anxiety, nor are they helpful alone for psychotic reactions. In mixed anxiety-depression they ought to be used with an antidepressant. They should not be prescribed during the first trimester of pregnancy. The following conditions may respond to these drugs.

Dysfunctional Anxiety

Ordinarily, they are given in brief courses of treatment, although exceptions exist. Expect a therapeutic response within a week after adequate dosage levels are reached. Patients with a history of alcoholism or drug dependence should not be given the benzodiazepines after the detoxification or withdrawal phase.

Muscle Spasm or Spasticity

Upper motor neuron spasticity due to paraplegia, multiple sclerosis, or tetanus may be helped.

Psychosomatic Disorders

For cardiac anxiety, beta blockers are preferred, or they can be used in conjunction with benzodiazepines.

Epilepsy

Intravenous diazepam is considered the treatment of choice for status epilepticus. Clonazepam is useful for petit mal variants.

Uncontrolled Aggressive Behavior

Certain patients who want assistance in controlling their episodes of uncontrolled violence could be helped by a benzodiazepine.

Preanesthetic

The benzodiazepines are often employed before surgical anesthesia because of their mild respiratory depressant effect, and the amnesia that accompanies parenteral use.

Amnesic Agents

During endoscopic examinations they provide relaxation and amnesia.

Phencyclidine Toxicity

Benzodiazepines are useful drugs in containing the violence of acute PCP reactions. Butyrophenones and phenothiazines can be tried, but they add to the anticholinergic toxicity of PCP.

Sedative Withdrawal

Chlordiazepoxide and diazepam have been commonly used in alcohol withdrawal, less frequently in hypnotic withdrawal.

Insomnia

Flurazepam, temazepam, and triazolam have specific indications for insomnia. Flurazepam decreases sleep latency and frequent awakenings, and increases sleep time. Sleep stages III and IV are decreased. Temazepam and triazolam are short-life hypnotics.

Night Terrors and Sleepwalking

Night terrors and sleepwalking are Stage IV sleep activities. Benzodiazepines diminish Stage IV sleep and are used for these sleep disorders.

Narcotic Potentiation

Benzodiazepines enhance the effect of narcotics administered for analgesia.

Severe Unavoidable Stress

When external stress cannot be altered by environmental manipulation, combined psychotherapy and a benzodiazepine may assist the patient to endure the situation.

Obsessive-Compulsive Disorders

Tricyclic antidepressants alone or in combination with a benzodiazepine may ameliorate the symptoms of disabling obsessive thinking and compulsive behavior patterns.

Recurrent Panic States

Disruptive panicky states that can include hyperventilation and tetany might be aborted by full doses of a benzodiazepine.

Phobic Anxiety

Phobias like agoraphobia may respond to desensitization techniques or amine oxidase inhibitors. If they do not, a course of benzodiazepines should be tried.

Some of the conditions listed above will require prolonged benzodiazepine therapy; for example, phobias, obsessive-compulsive states, muscle spasticity, and chronic panic states. Supervision of the patient is particularly necessary during their protracted use.

SIDE EFFECTS AND DRUG/BENZODIAZEPINES INTERACTIONS

Drowsiness is the most common of the unwanted effects. Weakness, fatigue, and slight difficulty in speaking may be noted. Ataxia is infrequent but should be particularly avoided in the elderly. Paradoxical irritability and rage are rare, and they seem to represent disinhibitory effects and some loss of ego controls. Depression can emerge during benzodiazepine therapy. The benzodiazepines have been used as drugs of abuse, usually as one of several drugs taken simultaneously.

The use of large amounts of caffeine will reduce the anxiolytic effect of the benzodiazepines. In fact, caffeine-containing beverages should be reduced or eliminated to determine whether caffeine constitutes the reason for the anxiety. Unlike the barbiturates, the benzodiazepines do not interfere with the action of other classes of drugs. It may be that tobacco use reduces the benzodiazepine effect and cimetidine (Tagamet) may increase it. When used as an anticonvulsant, diazepam is compatible with phenytoin (Dilantin).

HOW TO USE THE BENZODIAZEPINES

No psychotropic drug is so safe that it can be prescribed casually and without supervision. The benzodiazepines are not so safe that they can be prescribed for trivial indications or without proper supervision of the patient.

Ideally, if time is available, treatment should begin at low doses and gradually be increased to achieve satisfactory relief. The benzodiazepine is then gradually decreased so that the patient is functioning effectively without more than mild anxiety. These drugs work best when combined with counseling about methods of dealing with tension and stress. If long-term therapy is necessary, brief benzodiazepine holidays are interposed during periods of low stress.

When the drug is to be discontinued, it should be done gradually if full therapeutic doses have been used, particularly if they have been taken for months or years. The reduction should be the equivalent of 2 mg to 5 mg of diazepam weekly. Although millions of people have discontinued therapeutic amounts of benzodiazepines abruptly without difficulty, a few have experienced withdrawal symptoms. Not all symptoms following withdrawal are withdrawal symptoms. They may be re-emerging anxiety that had been contained with the benzodiazepine. These tend to increase in severity over time, but withdrawal symptoms tend to improve after seven to ten days following discontinuance.

REFERENCES

1. Cohen, S. The benzodiazepines. Psychiatric Annals. 13: 65-70, 1983.
2. Hines, L.R. Toxicology and side effects of anxiolytics. In: Handbook of Experimental Pharmacology, Vol. 55 IV, Ed.: F. Hoffmeiser. Springer Verlag, Berlin, 1981.
3. Snyder, S.H. Benzodiazepine receptors. Psychiatric Annals. 11: 19-23, 1981.
4. Hollister, L.E. Pharmacology and pharmacokinetics of the minor tranquilizers. Psychiatric Annals. 11: 26-31, 1981.

5. Kales, A., Scharf, M.B. and Kales, J.D. Science. 201: 1039, 1978.
6. Kales, A., Soldators, C. R., Bixler, E.O. and Kales, J.D. Early morning insomnia with rapidly eliminated benzodiazepines. Science. 220: 95-97, 1983.

28. Benzodiazepine Receptors in the Brain

The exciting recent discoveries of specific opioid receptor sites and of endogenous pain-relieving peptides, the endorphins and enkephalins, have opened up new lines of research into the chemistry and physiology of the brain.

Apparently, the naturally occurring analgesics do more than relieve pain. They modulate feeling tones and, perhaps, have significant roles to play in certain mental illnesses.

Another example of psychotherapeutic drugs acting on specific receptor sites are the antipsychotic agents. They block dopamine receptors in certain areas of the brain at the nucleus accumbens to exert their antipsychotic action, and in the extrapyramidal nucleii to produce movement disorders like Parkinsonism.

It was found and amply confirmed a few years ago that the benzodiazepines also bind to specific receptors on certain neuronal membranes near the synaptic junctions. Since the benzodiazepines are the most common of all prescribed drug groups, this finding is an important development. These drugs are considered to have anxiolytic, anticonvulsant, muscle relaxant, and hypnotic properties. Until the binding site discovery their mechanism of action was incompletely understood. They were assumed to have some sort of functional relationship to GABA and to glycine transmitters.

Just as the revelation that opiate receptors existed stimulated a search for some internal chemical that can fit onto them, a scrutiny of naturally occurring substances that might occupy the benzodiazepine site also is under way. Will an anxiety-reducing or convulsion threshold-elevating internal substance be found? It is quite likely, and already we have some hints about its nature.

NEUROPHYSIOLOGY OF THE RECEPTOR

Benzodiazepine binding sites are unevenly distributed in the central nervous system and are found in highest concentrations in the cerebral cortex, the cerebellum, and the amygdala, with fewer located in the hippocampus, thalamus, hypothalamus, spinal cord, and extrapyramidal nucleii. The medulla, pons, and corpus callosum have very few benzodiazepine receptors. This distribution is quite unlike the location of opioid receptors. Unlike opioid receptors that are also found in the gut, the benzodiazepine sites have been identified mainly in the brain and spinal cord with some evidence of specific kidney binding of the benzodiazepines.

As proof that these receptors have a specificity for the benzodiazepine molecule, Mohler and Okada and Squires and Braestrup independently established that the higher potency benzodiazepines bind to the receptors more firmly than lower potency benzodiazepines. Members of this class with high anticonvulsant activity, for example, are more tightly bound than those with lower antiseizure activity. When benzodiazepines are listed according to their clinical potency, the listing generally corresponds to their affinity for the receptor.

The benzodiazepine receptor is not positioned on dopamine norepinephrine, acetylcholine, or GABA nerve terminals. Benzodiazepines that occupy the site are not displaced by any of these neurotransmitters nor by histamine, serotonin, glutamate, glycine, asparate, substance P, or methenkepalin. Only the sterospecific benzodiazepines possess a substantial degree of activity on the receptor.

Up to now more than 100 nonbenzodiazepine psychotropic compounds, 14 putative neurotransmitters, and more than 100 peptides have exhibited either no affinity or only a low affinity for the benzodiazepine binding site.

Apparently, inhibition of benzodiazepine binding will occur with caffeine, theophyllin, and aminophyllin. The precise meaning of this inhibition is not apparent. There are also normally occurring purines that have been identified as inhibitors of benzodiazepine binding. They are inosine and hypoxanthine. Speculations that they may be the endogenous substances that normally occupy the benzodiazepine receptors have been suggested. If this turns out to be correct, their inhibition of binding would signify an occupation of the site prior to administration of the drug.

The two purines do increase the latency of Metrazol convulsions in rodents just as the benzodiazepines do. The fact that inosine and hypoxanthine have only an evanescent affinity for these receptors, however, casts some doubt upon their role as putative benzodiazepinoid transmitters. It has been determined, however, that only a small number of receptors need to be occupied in order to manifest anticonvulsive and antianxiety effects.

The receptor has been found in all vertebrates back to the bony fishes. In the more primitive fishes and in still lower species the benzodiazepine receptor is not detectable. Its presence has been confirmed in humans, where it becomes manifest shortly before birth and is developed to its maximal concentration about a week after birth.

The activity of the benzodiazepines as anticonvulsants is well established. It was therefore of interest to learn that the number of benzodiazepine receptors rapidly increased following experimentally induced generalized seizures in rats. The postictal increase in cortical benzodiazepine receptors indicates that the brain may be more sensitive to these drugs following seizures. In instances of status epilepticus an enhanced activity might be expected.

Diazepam is considered the drug of choice in recurrent seizure states. It is firmly established that the benzodiazepines inhibit certain types of neuronal transmission thereby reducing seizure and other excitatory activity. It will be interesting to see whether direct correlations exist between the anticonvulsant and the antianxiety effects of the various benzodiazepines because more than one type of receptor has been identified. An excellent correlation is present between the number of sites occupied by diazepam and its ability to protect against electrically induced or Metrazol seizures.

A strain of "nervous" mice has been bred that also have a selective loss of Purkinje cells in the cerebellum. When radio-labelled diazepam is injected into this mutant strain, a marked decrease in its uptake can be measured as compared with that of the normal (nonnervous) littermates. The Purkinje cells are believed to be important in the neurophysiological expression of the activity of benzodiazepines. Since their action is inhibitory, the firing of these cells dampens neuronal excitation. In patients dying of Huntington's disease, cerebellar benzodiazepine receptor cells are greatly diminished in number, and they show a loss of Purkinje cells at autopsy.

Up to now the assumption has been made that the benzodiazepines may act over serotonin, GABA, or glycine systems, particularly in view of their anticonvulsant activity. Some sort of relationship to GABA may exist, although it has been demonstrated that the receptors for this substance are in different locations from the benzodiazepine receptor. Among its other pharmacologic effects, benzodiazepines may function as GABA enhancers, since GABA dampens seizure activity. What benzodiazepines seem to do is to potentiate the inhibiting effects of GABA.

IMPLICATIONS

1. Does the human have built-in calming and/or anticonvulsant chemical substances? It would seem so, otherwise how can the presence of receptors that are benzodiazepine specific be explained? Since other antianxiety agents like the barbiturates and the propanediols (meprobamate-like drugs) act in a nonspecific manner in the brain, the benzodiazepines are unique in their binding to particular receptors. It may be found that other molecular entities also can attach to the benzodiazepine receptor. If so, it could be predicted that they either will have properties similar to the benzodiazepines or will act as antagonists by blockading the site.

2. It will be interesting to watch the further development of this discovery. For example, are nondrug techniques for anxiety reduction like relaxation or meditation mediated through the internal chemical that fits onto the benzodiazepine site?

3. Another clinical implication may be derived. These drugs should be gradually rather than abruptly discontinued after prolonged use in order to give the endogenous ligand the opportunity to increase and reoccupy the receptors.

4. Is it possible that we will find a subgroup of chronically anxious people who have a constitutional absence or diminished level of the endogenous antianxiety or anticonvulsant substance, or a congenitally reduced number of the specific receptors?

5. It is tempting to predict that severe situational stress will cause an increased requirement for the internal ligand that fits onto the benzodiazepine receptor site.

SUMMARY

The fascinating discovery of yet another specific receptor site in the central nervous system that can be occupied by psychotropic compounds of the benzodiazepine group may foreshadow important theoretical and practical information about brain function. It is interesting that all three of the therapeutic drug classes that act on receptors—the opiates, the antipsychotics, and the benzodiazepines—all inhibit neuronal transmission. Nerve cell inhibition appears to be at least as important as excitation in the brain's work.

BIBLIOGRAPHY

- Braestrup, C. and Squires, R.F. Brain specific benzodiazepine receptors. Brit. J. Psychiat. 133:249-260, 1978.
- Mohler, H. and Okada, T. Benzodiazepine receptor: Demonstration in the central nervous system. Science. 198:849-851, 1977.
- Mohler, H. and Okada, T. The benzodiazepine receptor in human brain. In: Sleep Research, Eds.: R.G. Priest, A. Pletscher and J. Ward. MEP Press, 1979, pp. 3-12.
- Paul, S.M. and Skolnick, P. Rapid changes in brain benzodiazepine receptors after experimental seizures. Science. 202:891-892, 1978
- Skolnick, P. et al. CNS benzodiazepines receptors: Physiological studies and putative endogenous ligands. Pharmacology Biochemistry and Behavior. 10:815-823, 1979.
- Squires, R.F. and Braestrup, C. Benzodiazepine receptors in rat brain. Nature. 266:732-734, 1977.

29. Caffeine

The most widely used of all mind-altering drugs is, of course, caffeine. It is a remarkably safe substance—except for those sensitive to its effects and those who consume large quantities.

In this country it is ingested most frequently as coffee (85–150 mg per cup). Tea contains about half as much caffeine, and cola drinks have about a third as much per serving. It is present in many analgesics, being the "C" in APCs. Excedrin is formulated with 65 mg of caffeine. Other over-the-counter preparations in which caffeine may be found include antiobesity, stimulant, and decongestant nostrums. To demonstrate the extent of its usage, this country imported over 4 billion dollars worth of coffee last year.

WHAT DOES CAFFEINE DO?

As a mild stimulant, caffeine is said to or has been shown to decrease fatigue, elevate mood mildly, and improve alertness and work output. Reaction time decreases and drowsiness may lessen. Thinking is either unchanged or accelerated slightly. The coffee break has become an established institution indicating, perhaps, that worker efficiency improves with coffee. However, the brief period of work cessation may also contribute to any enhanced performance following the break. Most users are unaware of any change in their psychological state. Others may generally feel better.

WHERE MAY CAFFEINE BE FOUND?

Table 29–1 indicates the common and infrequent sources of caffeine (modified from Greden).

HOW DOES CAFFEINE DO IT?

A note in *Science* (211:1408-1409, 1981) supports the significance of the purine adenosine in explaining caffeine's action. Adenosine depresses neuro-

Table 29–1
Caffeine Content of Common Drinks and Proprietary Medicines

Coffee	85–150 mg per cup
Tea	50–100 mg per cup
Decaffeinated coffee	2–4 mg per cup
Cola drinks	40–50 mg per 12-oz glass
Cocoa	5–20 mg per cup
Chocolate bar, small	15–25 mg per bar
No Doz	100 mg per dosage unit
Vivarin	200 mg per dosage unit
Anacin	32.5 mg per dosage unit
APC	32 mg per dosage unit
Bromoseltzer	35.5 mg per dosage unit
Cafergot	100 mg per dosage unit
Comeback	100 mg per dosage unit
Darvon Compound	32 mg per dosage unit
Empirin Compound	32 mg per dosage unit
Excedrin	64.8 mg per dosage unit
Fiorinal	40 mg per dosage unit
Pre-Mens	66 mg per dosage unit
Vanquish	32 mg per dosage unit

Modified from Greden, *Psychosomatics* 21:418, 1980.

nal firing in many brain areas by retarding the release of biogenic amines. This is antagonized by caffeine occupying adenosine binding sites on the brain cell, preventing adenosine's CNS depressant action. The net result is increased firing and psychic stimulation. The theory that caffeine works by inhibiting phosphodiesterase which breaks down cyclic AMP (adenosine monophosphate) seems less likely.

WHY DO PEOPLE DRINK COFFEE?

The widespread use of coffee tends to induce adolescents and other nonusers to develop the habit. Family and peer examples must be an important influence. As a cultural tradition of hospitality often associated with other pleasant activities (conversation, relaxation), it becomes a rewarding pastime. Much socializing centers around tea or coffee. Its odor and taste may be attractive to some, but these are not strong motivations. Of course, the stimulant effects are sought after, especially by workers under pressure. Eventually, however, as tolerance develops, these are not marked, and the conditioned behavior is as likely to be as causative as the pharmacological action.

DOES CAFFEINE HAVE ANY MEDICAL USEFULNESS?

The use of medicinal caffeine has diminished in recent years. It probably has no direct analgesic effect. Instead, the mild mood elevation may account for any pain-relieving quality it may possess. It is no longer employed in the treatment of depressant drug overdose. Caffeine has been tried in the hyperkinetic behavioral disorders of children with varying results. As an anorexiant, its value is doubtful, unless large amounts are taken. The only value it may have in decongestant formulations is to counteract the sedative action of antihistamines.

Caffeine has been combined with ergot as Cafergot for migraine. Its rationale for this purpose may be its mild vasoconstrictive action on cerebral blood vessels. It is widely used to recover from alcohol intoxication (why the coffee has to be black remains unknown). Certain symptoms of alcohol intoxication are reversed, but not all—hand steadiness, for example. Coffee is also generally taken for the drowsiness associated with prolonged driving. It may be effective, but just as important is breaking up the prolonged driving period.

HAS DEATH DUE TO CAFFEINE OVERDOSE
EVER BEEN RECORDED?

Fatalities due to caffeine poisoning are extremely rare. The few deaths that have been reported were preceded by excitement, delirium, light flashes, and tinnitus. Tachycardia, extrasystoles, and hyperpnea occur. Seizures are a possibility. A definite lethal dose cannot be stated, but may be approximately 10 grams. Theophylline, a related compound (caffeine is trimethylxanthine and theophylline is dimethylxanthine), has been much more frequently involved in overdose deaths. The rapid intravenous use of therapeutic amounts of aminophyllin (a theophyllin-ethylenediamine complex) has been associated with sudden death.

WHAT ABOUT CAFFEINE AND FETAL DAMAGE?

At usual levels of coffee drinking genetic changes do not occur. It is possible that pregnant women who drink more than six cups of coffee a day are at greater risk to have spontaneous abortions or stillbirths. Pregnant women who are double digit coffee drinkers should be advised to moderate their caffeine intake during pregnancy.

WHAT IS CAFFEINE INTOXICATION?

DSM III includes a diagnosis of caffeine intoxication. It accompanies the chronic use of large amounts of caffeine-containing products, 750 mg or more a day. The manifestations include nausea, insomnia, restlessness, jitteryness, and other symptoms simulating anxiety. Muscle twitching, diuresis, a flushed face, and psychomotor agitation are sometimes present. Palpitations and extrasystoles can occur. Since caffeine stimulates gastric acid secretion, exacerbations of peptic ulcers are possible. At very high doses grand mal convulsions have been described. This is caffeinism as described by Greden who obtained high scores in such individuals on anxiety rating scales. They also tend to use more anxiolytics and hypnosedatives than non-coffee drinkers or moderate coffee drinkers.

Caffeinism is also possible in those people sensitive to this drug. A single cup of coffee may produce undesired wakefulness, nervousness, diarrhea, nausea, and vomiting. For those hypersensitive individuals caffeine is a toxic substance. On the other hand there are others who appear able to swallow enormous amounts of coffee without obvious difficulty.

Greden recommends confirming the diagnosis by a program of gradual withdrawal over a period of a week or two. The complaints will diminish, sometimes dramatically. If necessary, a caffeine challenge is employed. The patient is permitted to resume the intake of caffeine. The return of the symptoms is likely. The patient is again detoxified. This procedure should convince both patient and doctor of the cause of the complaints.

WHAT ABOUT TOLERANCE AND
AN ABSTINENCE SYNDROME?

Tolerance certainly occurs. In fact, the low medicinal use of caffeine may have come about because of the nation's tolerance to the drug. People who drink coffee all day have a high degree of tolerance. Those who develop the difficult-to-diagnose syndrome of caffeine intoxication have exceeded their partial tolerance.

When the intake of caffeine is abruptly discontinued in chronically tolerant consumers, a withdrawal syndrome may emerge within 24 hours.

Even the "let down" feeling 4 to 6 hours after the last cup may be a prodromal symptom of withdrawal. It is more than likely that the individual who is unable to function after a night's rest until the day's first cup of coffee has been downed, is treating an abstinence syndrome. Headache is a key symptom. It is described as throbbing and diffuse. Irritability, lethargy, and yawning are often seen. A cup of coffee will relieve the headache and so will a caffeine-containing patent medicine. Unless the diagnosis is made, the cycle of caffeinism and caffeine withdrawal tends to recur.

HOW IS CAFFEINISM TREATED?

A greater problem than treatment is diagnosis. Caffeinism is not considered and is often called anxiety, anxiety-depression, or some mimicking condition. After diagnosis and education of the patient, a gradual detoxification should be done. The substitution of equivalent activities ought to be instituted. Noncaffeine-containing drinks, including decaffeinated coffee, are recommended.

CAN A HEAVY COFFEE DRINKER BECOME A MODERATE DRINKER?

It would be preferable for those who have had a number of troublesome experiences with caffeine to abandon its use completely. Practically, this does not always happen after the symptoms of caffeinism have remitted. Some former caffeinists are able to moderate their usage. Others tend to escalate to previous levels of caffeine intake and develop evidence of caffeine intoxication again.

SUMMARY

Despite its evident safety, caffeine can be harmful to those hypersensitive to its effects and those who overuse the substance. This repeats the oft-told tale: No drug is completely safe, not even the ubiquitous cup of coffee or tea.

It is difficult for the clinician to consider that caffeine-containing beverages and medicines might be the cause of the symptoms the patient is presenting. This is especially true if the physician has a bubbling pot of coffee on the desk. But it may be so.

BIBLIOGRAPHY

- Farkas, C.S. Caffeine intake and potential effect on health of a segment of northern Canadian indigenous people. Int. J. Addictions. 14: 27-43, 1979.

- Greden, J.F. Anxiety or caffeinism: A diagnostic dilemma. Am. J. Psychiat. 131: 1089-1092, 1974.
- Greden, J.F. et al. Anxiety and depression associated with caffeinism among psychiatric inpatients. Am. J. Psychiat. 135: 963-966, 1978.
- Greden, J.F. et al. Caffeine-withdrawal headache: A clinical profile. Psychosomatics. 21: 411-418, 1980.
- Greden, J.F. Caffeine and tobacco dependence. In: *Comprehensive Textbook of Psychiatry*. Eds.: H. I. Kaplan, A. M. Freedman & B. J. Sadock. Williams & Wilkins, Baltimore, 1980.

30. Codeine Use and Abuse

The analgesic and soporific effects of opium derive from the approximately 10 percent of morphine it contains. However, other important alkaloids are present in opium, of which codeine (methylmorphine) is found in amounts of about 0.5 percent. Opium also contains a small amount of thebaine (dimethylmorphine) which is used to manufacture codeine.

CODEINE USE

For a century and a half codeine has been widely used as an analgesic and cough suppressant, and an enormous clinical experience has accrued. It has the reputation of being the safe narcotic when used in therapeutic amounts. The pain-relieving ratio of codeine to morphine is 120 mg to 10 mg when given subcutaneously, but the ratio is more favorable to codeine when they are taken by mouth. It is best used in combination with acetaminophen (Tylenol) or aspirin (codeine combinations) because these peripheral analgesics definitely add to the effect of the central action of codeine. Doses of 30 mg of codeine have been shown to be superior to a placebo in patients with a variety of painful conditions. In one study a dose of 15 mg of codeine plus 300 mg of aspirin was significantly more effective than 300 mg of aspirin alone.

Codeine combinations are effective for moderate pain. Increasing the dosage above 120 mg usually will not eliminate severe pain. This ceiling dose is also manifested by the emergence of side effects when codeine is taken in larger than therapeutic amounts. The undesirable symptoms include dizziness, nausea and vomiting, and sometimes irritability.

The intravenous use of codeine is not recommended. A histamine reaction is almost invariable, resulting in a flush, headache, hypotension, and hives. Sporadic attempts to inject the codeine combinations into a vein by persons abusing the combination have produced severe inflammatory reactions of the vein and, sometimes, pulmonary emboli.

Codeine cough syrups have traditionally been the standard antitussives, and they remain the drug of choice for cough suppression. The usual dose is 10 mg, but this may have to be exceeded or frequent dosing practiced. The nonnarcotic, dextromethorphan, which has little dependency-producing ability, has partially supplanted codeine cough preparations.

It is worth remembering that about 10 percent of codeine is excreted as morphine. Therefore a positive urine for both codeine and morphine may indicate codeine use alone, or codeine and morphine, or codeine and heroin use (heroin is rapidly transformed to morphine in the liver.)

CODEINE DEPENDENCE

Primary codeine dependence, in which codeine is the drug of choice, is a rarity. Codeine has a low binding affinity for the opiate receptor sites, and the euphoria is of low grade quality, not highly valued by opiate dependent people. This and the unpleasant side effects when large amounts are consumed explain why it is so infrequently preferred over other narcotics.

Secondary codeine dependence that occurs when heroin or other opiates become unavailable, is seen more often. During a heroin "panic" codeine cough syrups containing 10 mg per teaspoonful were commonly substituted. An old favorite was the elixir of terpin hydrate with codeine, perhaps because it also contained about 40 percent alcohol. It was not uncommon for a narcotic addict to drink four ounces of the codeine cough syrup four to six times a day in order to avoid the withdrawal reaction from heroin. Codeine can partially suppress the heroin abstinence syndrome.

In the usual therapeutic doses codeine had a low propensity to produce tolerance and withdrawal effects even when taken over protracted periods. Halpern,[1,2] director of the pain clinic at the University of Washington, has stated, "Prolonged use of codeine in the dosage of 65 mg every four to six hours for several months is associated with little risk of significant narcotic dependence. Tolerance does develop, however, requiring an increase in dosage to provide continuing relief. The low incidence of abuse should be contrasted with the frequent use and easy availability of the drug to dispel addiction-abuse fears."

In his review article Beaver[3] has noted, "While all narcotics possess the ability to induce physical dependence on prolonged administration, oral codeine has substantially less ability in this regard than such drugs as hycodone [Hycodan], oxycodone [Percodan], and meperidine [Demerol]."

A common clinical observation is that after sudden withdrawal from therapeutic amounts of codeine no or only minimal withdrawal symptoms are observed even after months of continuous treatment. In one experiment humans were given 130 mg of codeine daily for three months. After a challenge dose of Nalline, no abstinence symptoms appeared.

Jaffe[4] writes, "Although codeine can partially suppress morphine withdrawal, withdrawal symptoms after codeine (120–1800 mg/day), while qualitatively similar to those of morphine, are considerably less intense."

The codeine abuse situation is unusual in one respect. As a rule, widespread use of euphoriant drugs is predictive that they will be widely abused, if only on the basis of availability. This is not the pattern for codeine. Less than 1 percent of all narcotic addicts under treatment mention codeine as their drug of choice. In DAWN[5] mentions for 1981, codeine ranked 34th in emergency room mentions. Denmark has the highest codeine consumption per capita of any country for which records are kept. In a State Department report for 1981 on Denmark's drug abuse problem, codeine is not even mentioned.

DORS AND FOURS

Nevertheless even a drug with a lesser abuse potential like codeine can be abused, and some recent observations in this regard will be described.

The simultaneous use of multiple substances has emerged as a significant problem during the past 15 years. While the "speedball" (cocaine and heroin) is of more ancient vintage, the practice called polydrug abuse has expanded to the point that single drug abusers now seem to be in the minority. At times the array of mind-altering substances that are consumed is mind-boggling to both the consumer and the observer. At other times polydrug abuse has a specific intent: to enhance one drug's effects, to neutralize some undesired side effect of the primary drug, or to achieve a "high" less expensively by combining a smaller amount of some expensive agent with a cheaper substance.

Some favored combinations include methaqualone (Quaalude) and alcohol, and barbiturates with alcohol, but marijuana and alcohol combinations are probably the most common drug mixtures of all. The oral narcotic analgesics participate in the polydrug abuse phenomenon. Propoxyphene (Darvon) is used with a variety of tranquilizers and sedatives. Pentazocine (Talwin) and pyribenzamine (Ts and blues) are a favorite in a number of midwestern cities. Its intravenous use is widespread enough so that the manufacturer of Talwin has incorporated the narcotic antagonist, naloxone (Narcan), in the Talwin formulation to neutralize the narcotic effect if it is used intravenously, but not to interfere with its oral use.

In Southern California "loads" or "dors and fours"—glutethimide (Doriden) and codeine #4—have become a more recent addition to the polydrug list. Doriden is a sleeping pill. Codeine #4 contains 65 mg of codeine with 300 mg of either aspirin or Tylenol. The preferred "load" recipe consists of two codeine #4 and one 50 mg Doriden tablet. The usual amount swallowed (only rarely injected) is four codeine #4 and two Doriden tablets, but tolerant individuals are capable of consuming much larger amounts.

That this combination is hazardous is attested to by the fact that two-thirds of the nation's codeine-related deaths have occurred in Southern California during 1981.[5] At present it appears that "dors and fours" are being used by fewer people, not so much because the combination can be lethal, but because the sources of supply have been sharply reduced. A number of "stress clinics" and private physicians whose practice consisted of prescribing the ingredients to make "loads" and similar concoctions have been closed down and prosecuted.

It seems that the current poor quality of the heroin (2 to 5 percent) is the reason for the switch to less satisfying narcotics. When a drug like codeine is combined with a hypnosedative like Doriden, the depressant effects on the brain are intensified. The user feels distanced from anxieties and frustrations. When such people are observed, they seem to be in a toxic delirium with confusion, loss of control over behavior, speech slurring, ataxia, amnesia, and "nodding out." A number of car and other types of accidents have been traced to the narcotic-sedative combinations. After being on these drug mixtures for weeks or months, sudden discontinuance produces an abstinence syndrome reminiscent of sedative-hypnotic withdrawal, including convulsions.

Treatment consists of support of vital functions, anticonvulsants and a trial of naloxone (Narcan), which antagonizes the respiratory depression that codeine can induce. It will not improve the respiratory depressant action of Doriden. At times the large amount of aspirin or acetaminophen that is taken will induce gastrointestinal or hepatic disturbances.

SUMMARY

General agreement exists that oral codeine in combination with a peripheral analgesic like aspirin or Tylenol will ameliorate moderate pain satisfactorily. Despite its low potential for abuse when used alone, codeine has had a recent vogue in combination with Doriden for purposes of intoxication.

Supplies of the two components of "loads" have come from inordinate prescription writing by physicians or clinics writing for profit. Thus, the Southern California "epidemic" can be considered as much a physician problem as a drug problem. Prompt identification and prosecution of the physicians and clinic owners have led to a decrease in the number of casualties seen.

REFERENCES

1. Halpern, L.M. Treating pain with drugs. Minnesota Med. March, 1974, pp. 176-184.

2. Halpern, L.M. and Bonica, J.J. Analgesics. In: *Drugs of Choice* 1980-1981, Ed.: W. Modell, St. Louis, Mosby, 1980.
3. Beaver, W.T. Mild analgesics: A review of their clinical pharmacology. Amer. J. Med. Sci. 250:577-603 (Nov) 1965.
4. Jaffe, J. Drug addiction and drug abuse. In: *The Pharmacological Basis of Therapeutics,* VI Edition, Eds.: A.G. Gilman, L.S. Goodman, and A. Gilman, New York, Macmillan, 1980.
5. N.I.D.A. Statistical Series, 1981 Data from the Drug Abuse Warning Network (DAWN) Series I, Number 1, 1982.

31. Paregoric

Paregoric (camphorated tincture of opium) has been used in medicine for over two centuries, mostly for the simple diarrheas of children. In addition to opium it contains camphor, benzoic acid, oil of anise, alcohol, and glycerin—all unnecessary for the reduction of bowel hypermotility.

Even the first edition (1940) of Goodman and Gilman's *Pharmacologic Basis of Therapeutics* noted that it represents "a needlessly complex therapeutic survival of a former day." This statement remains true 45 years later.

The camphor content may be downright harmful in predisposed children for it has been known to produce central nervous system symptoms including epileptiform convulsions. The active component is powdered opium, 400 mg in 100 ml. Since opium contains about 10 percent morphine, 40 mg morphine plus lesser amounts of codeine and other alkaloids are present in about three ounces of paregoric. Until 1970 camphorated tincture of opium was sold over the counter in most states. When the Controlled Substances Act became effective in 1971, it was placed in Schedule III and automatically required a prescription thereafter.

ABUSE HISTORY

Paregoric has an interesting and instructive history as an item of abuse. In those states where it was available over the counter before 1971, it was a significant abuse problem, particularly among the impoverished Black male populations. It was possible to obtain unlimited supplies simply by going from pharmacy to pharmacy and purchasing a couple of ounces from each. It was only required that the buyer be older than 18, have some sort of identification, and sign a register. Forty-eight hours later it was legal to return again for another bottle of tr. opiivcamph.

In many cities during the 1950s, paregoric was a very popular medicament, and not for diarrhea. Cities such as St. Louis, Miami, and Detroit had more paregoric addicts than heroin addicts. It was swallowed in large quantities, but even more frequent was its intravenous injection. In order to prepare paregoric for injection it was heated and flamed to burn off the alcohol and to evaporate most of the water. After cooling, the camphor floated to the top and could be skimmed off.

It was then filtered through absorbent cotton. Up to a quart of paregoric might be used in a single day. Such an amount contained about 400 mg of morphine base, equivalent to 150 mg to 200 mg of heroin. This represented a substantial habit, since the average amount in a present day "bag" varies from 5 to 20 mg of heroin. With the passage of the more restrictive Federal legislation in 1970, paregoric dependence practically disappeared, and it is a rarity these days.

COMPLICATIONS OF IV PAREGORIC USE

Three unhappy consequences of parenteral paregoric use were seen. The injected material was exceedingly irritant to the tissues at the site where it was instilled. Some of the worst inflammatory reactions and scarring ever observed in opiate addicts occurred in paregoric-dependent individuals. After the antecubital, saphenous, femoral, and other accessible veins had been occluded, the jugular vein and even the carotid artery were used. In those days it was possible to make a diagnosis of paregoric addiction by simply seeing a large, irregular, ugly scar on the neck overlying the great vessels.

The second complication occurred as the result of the occasional addition of Pyribenzamine (tripenelamine) to the injected paregoric. This mixture, called blue velvet, contained talcum, an insoluble filler material in Pyribenzamine, so that its intravenous infusion produced small emboli of the pulmonary vessels. Pulmonary hypertension, granulomas, and fibrosis resulted from chronic usage.

Finally, infections accompanying the unsterile injections seemed to develop at least as frequently with paregoric as with heroin and perhaps more often because it was filtered through less than sterile absorbent cotton. Abcesses, cellulitis, and thrombophlebitis were routinely encountered. Hepatitis, bacterial endocarditis, and septicemia were far from uncommon.

SIGNIFICANCE OF THE PAREGORIC DECADE

We hear so little about paregoric these days that its abuse not too long ago tends to be forgotten. Those who cared for the sick people remember their high mortality from pulmonary insufficiency and infections. Another memory is of the dozens, sometimes hundreds, of empty paregoric bottles littering the streets and alleys not too far from the drug stores where the paregoric had been purchased.

Why do we not have a paregoric problem now? It seems that simply making the concoction more difficult to obtain was sufficient to eliminate the problem. If so, it represents one of the major successes of the Controlled Substances Act of 1970.

The lesson to be learned from the paregoric story is that availability is a prime factor in the initiation and perpetuation of substance-abusing behavior. Fifteen years ago paregoric was the cheapest and most readily available of the opiates, and when it became more difficult to acquire, paregoric addiction vanished. What remains unknown is the subsequent fate of the paregoric mainliners. Some may have gone over to heroin use, but others undoubtedly stopped using opiates.

When plentiful supplies of an inexpensive intoxicant are easily obtained, it is impossible to deter its usage. This is the lesson of penny gin in eighteenth-century England, of laudanum in nineteenth-century England, of opium smoking prior to the Opium Wars in China, and of coca paste smoking in present-day Peru. It accounts for the etheromania in certain counties in Ireland over a hundred years ago, the large-scale sniffing of shoemakers' glue in the prison in Monterrey, Mexico, and for many other epidemics of intoxicant abuse by a large portion of the exposed population.

Although availability is a major element determining which substance will be abused, it does not mean that the interdiction of that substance will therefore bring an end to the problem of drug abuse. So many other mind-altering substances are at hand that many consumers will switch to one of the others. However, all abusable natural and synthetic chemicals should be made as difficult to come by as possible. Many consumers become discouraged as drugs become more difficult for them to obtain.

The goal of a complete elimination of all abused drugs from a society is difficult to achieve in a social system like ours. A more realistic objective would be for a partial reduction, making procurement more difficult and more costly. An even better solution would consist of a decrease in demand as a result of educational-preventive-treatment measures that increase the resistance of young and old to indulgence in abusive drug taking.

Since there was no marked increase in heroin or other opiate addiction after certain states (like Michigan in 1965) stopped over-the-counter (OTC) sales of paregoric, it appears that a number of users did clean up. Therefore, wise legislation can do some good, just as unwise legislation, such as not controlling Quaalude for a few years after it was introduced, can do harm.

RECENT DEVELOPMENTS

A recommendation that paregoric be permitted to be sold over the counter has surfaced again. It is claimed that an effective medication for simple diarrhea cannot be purchased without a prescription. The kaolin-pectin mixtures are said not to be effective. In addition to a predictable repetition of our unhappy experience with paregoric dependence, such a move is unwise for other reasons.

The camphor content in paregoric is capable of causing convulsive episodes in children, and there is no therapeutic rationale in the mixture. If it were to be removed, it would simply increase the ease with which paregoric can be converted into an injectable agent.

A second objection to relaxing the prescription requirement for paregoric is that most pediatricians do not believe that decreasing the motility of the bowel is proper treatment for infantile diarrhea. They recommend replacement fluids and electrolytes as needed, along with general supportive measures.

It has been amply demonstrated that those who do not remember history are condemned to repeat it. The disappearance of paregoric dependency is one of our few notable successes against opiate dependence. To lightly return to the past situation of easy access to this drug would be a public health blunder. Surely we are capable of developing alternative OTC antidiarrheal preparations without reviving paregoric.

Even if we are unable to do so, proprietary preparations of kaolin, pectin, and paregoric are sold OTC at present. They contain less paregoric per dose and the pectin and kaolin make it impossible to produce an injectable preparation from them. These formulations hardly can be abused when taken by mouth, and the amount of paregoric obtained discourages nonmedical use. Because of this, they should be satisfactory antidiarrheal concoctions for those who believe that some degree of bowel motility reduction is desirable.

TREATMENT OF NEONATAL OPIATE WITHDRAWAL

Paregoric doses of 2 to 10 drops per kg body weight every four hours retain therapeutic usefulness in the withdrawal of infants born to opiate-dependent mothers. It should be used for two to four weeks and gradually discontinued. Although paregoric is the opiate preparation generally used because of its long tradition in the management of opioid dependence in the neonate, tincture of opium would be just as effective and a bit more rational. Other drugs used for this purpose include appropriately small amounts of chlorpromazine, phenobarbital, diazepam, and methadone. Clonidine has not yet been tried for neonatal opiate addiction, but it may be effective in view of its success in the adult opiate withdrawal syndrome.

SUMMARY

Since a real danger exists of its diversion to support an opiate type of dependency, paregoric should not become an OTC preparation again. In addition, its indication as an antidiarrheal for children is no longer generally accepted, and the neurotoxicity of camphor may be hazardous. Thus, little or no basis exists for changing the current legal status of paregoric. Indeed, it would be a short-sighted, perilous venture to do so.

BIBLIOGRAPHY

- Burton, J. F. et al. Mainliners and blue velvet, J. Forensic Sci. 10:466, 1965.
- Lerner, A. M. The abuse of paregoric in Detroit, Michigan (1956-1965). Bull. Narcotics. 18:31 (Jul-Sept) 1966.
- Oesther, F. J. et al. Infections in paregoric addicts. JAMA 190: 683 (Nov 16) 1964.
- Reddy, A. M. et al. Observations on heroin and methadone withdrawal in the newborn. Pediatrics. 48:353 (Sept) 1971.

32. The Rise and Fall of the Look-Alikes

Supply control is an essential aspect of drug abuse control. However, when demand reduction does not take place at the same time, consumers will transfer their usage to other items no matter how inferior. A few years ago we witnessed the emergence of such a phenomenon. It was a bizarre outgrowth of the Controlled Substances Act of 1970. This statute was an effort to reduce supplies of certain prescription drugs. Since the law was made operational, the quota for legally manufactured amphetamines was reduced by 80 percent. At the same time, the counterfeiting of amphetamines came under somewhat better control.

The unfilled demand for stimulants was perceived by an enterprising trucker in Florida who obtained a quantity of phenylpropanolamine (PPA), ephedrine, and caffeine tablets made to look like Dexedrine and other prescription stimulants. He proceeded to sell them whenever he arrived at a truck stop. Business became so good that a nationwide distribution system was set up. Other me-too entrepreneurs rushed in to share in the profits. At the height of the look-alike period, dozens of manufacturers and hundreds of "speed" boutiques were actively distributing stimulant look-alikes.

As could be predicted, the look-alikes expanded to "downer" look-alikes and to cocaine mimickers. The sales pitch was that these copycat drugs were safe, less expensive, and legal. Some stores dealt exclusively in the look-alike, sound-alike business. Others took them in as profitable sidelines.

The look-alikes contained drugs found in over-the-counter medications, but usually in larger amounts in order to provide greater potency. They mimicked "cartwheels" (amphetamine sulfate), "rainbows" (Tuinal), or "black beauties" (Biphetamine) among other bogus brands.

By 1981 millions of doses were being made and profits to the industry were estimated at 50 million dollars a year. Eventually, a multimedia campaign including direct mail advertising, ads in certain magazines, handbills in classrooms and at truckstops, and signs on campus bulletin boards proclaimed the availability of hassle-free mood changers.

Confronted by this propaganda barrage aimed at adolescents and adults alike, pressure from parent groups and other organizations built up to stop these "practice" drugs which many saw as an easy step on the road to the more potent agents. Post office seizures were made, and local and state ordinances prohibiting look-alike sales were enacted. The FDA declared that combinations of PPA, ephedrine, and caffeine constituted a new drug and would require federal approval before marketing. This did not affect the proprietary drugs sold without a prescription because none of them contained all three stimulants together. Misbranding and mislabeling were charged against some outlet owners. For example, one cocaine look-alike was labeled as an incense, not to be used for medical purposes. Most states have prohibitive legislation passed or pending.

How harmful are the look-alikes? When ordinary doses are taken, they are rarely dangerous. However, if used to achieve a "high," about four to eight dosage units must be consumed, and then the risks mount. Increasing numbers of complications are being reported.

The components of the various look-alikes will be described along with their possible untoward effects.

THE AMPHETAMINE LOOK-ALIKES

They have been combinations of the three drugs already mentioned, although the FDA ruling may reduce them to one or two.

1. Phenylpropanolamine

Usually present in 25 to 50 mg amounts. PPA has an ephedrine-like action, reducing appetite and producing alerting and mild stimulation. People with hypertension or coronary artery disease should not use the compound. In larger than average amounts dizziness, tremulousness, anxiety, palpitations, and nausea can occur. Sudden, marked rises in blood pressure have resulted in cerebral hemorrhages, according to a few published cases. A PPA psychosis has been described when large doses are consumed by vulnerable people. A regulatory discussion is under way concerning PPA. It may be made a prescription item because of its potential for harm when used under unsupervised conditions.

2. Ephedrine

The look-alikes usually contain from 12.5 to 50 mg. Ephedrine increases norepinephrine activity by increasing adrenergic receptor sensitivity. As a stimulant it is about five times weaker than amphetamine. It increases blood pressure and heart rate and dilates bronchioles. The same precautions and side effects hold for ephedrine as for PPA.

3. Caffeine

The caffeine content in the look-alikes ranges from 37.5 to 325 mg; the latter amount is about the same as three cups of strong coffee. People who are sensitive to caffeine, or those who use large amounts, are aware that headache, jitteriness, palpitations, anxiety, and gastritis can occur. Enormous doses are capable of producing convulsions and heart rhythm disturbances. The lethal dose of caffeine is said to be about 10 grams, or about 30 of the high dose, look-alike tablets.

These three substances are considered to be mild stimulants, but when taken together, additive effects will occur, and what was mild can become severe.

THE COCAINE LOOK-ALIKES

The concoctions are flakes or powders that resemble cocaine and may provide some stimulation on inhalation. More than a dozen products of variable content are known, including Peruvian Flake, Pseudocaine, Snocaine, Toot, Florida Snow, Real Caine, and Ultra Caine. The active ingredients may include ephedrine, PPA, caffeine, procaine, benzocaine, lidocaine, or related drugs. Lidocaine is more likely to produce cardiac arrest in some people than cocaine. In addition to their sale in shops or mail order establishments, they are sometimes sold as cocaine on the street. These look-alike, sound-alike products are sold to youths as practice cocaine.

THE SEDATIVE-HYPNOTIC LOOK-ALIKES

Most of the sedating look-alikes contain 25 to 50 mg of the antihistamine doxylamine succinate, also found in proprietaries like Formula 44 and Nyquill. Many formulations contain an analgesic like acetaminophen (Tylenol) or salicylamide, an aspirin-like compound. The use of alcohol with such look-alikes can induce oversedation. Doxylamine overdose is associated with confusion, tremors, and stupor.

Quaaludes (methaqualone) remain popular among chemical hedonists. Therefore they are widely counterfeited. Many of the Quaalude-appearing tablets stamped "Lemmon 714" contain no methaqualone. Phenobarbital and diazepam are the common adulterants. Some street Quaalude tablets on analysis have been found to have 200 mg of diazepam, about 40 times the average dose of that drug. The look-alike Quaaludes contain doxylamine succinate and resemble the real thing in appearance.

COMMENT

Have the look-alikes served any useful purpose? It appears not. Even when used as an aid to cram for exams or to drive a truck through the night, stimulants have not been shown to be effective. While they admittedly diminish drowsiness, they do not improve mental or motor functioning. The user is awake, tired, perhaps jittery, and with decreased cognitive abilities. The trucker's occupational hallucinations often are based upon stimulant-generated misperceptions. Truck accidents occur both when driving while drowsy and when fatigued but awake following stimulant use.

Have the look-alikes had adverse public health consequences? They have. They have been promoted among and used by school children. This establishes nonmedical drug-using patterns early in life. Juveniles start using these "drugs for kids" in their constant search for peer admiration. The move to the real thing becomes an easier decision. The major prevention axiom: "Don't pollute your body with any substance that is unneeded" is undermined by look-alike propaganda.

These drugs are not safe when ingested in the amounts necessary to achieve euphoria. At the dosages needed to obtain an amphetamine or barbiturate effect, they have as many dangers as the amphetamines and barbiturates.

The point to be learned from the look-alike caper is that control of supplies, important as it is, is not enough. In a modern society there are always substitutes or analogues to be found, or chemists who will make them, and citizens who will deal in them. At the same time that strenuous interdiction efforts are undertaken, the populations at risk must be helped to understand why nontherapeutic drug taking is eventually counterproductive. We are properly concerned about the external pollutants in the environment. It is a matter of greater concern when internal pollutants are introduced into that unique but delicate organ, the brain.

SUMMARY

It seems that we may be seeing the end of the look-alike episode. But man's ability to exploit his fellows should never be underestimated. Without wise countermeasures, some chemical equivalent will rise again.

BIBLIOGRAPHY

- California Society for Treatment and Other Drug Dependencies News. Stimulant Look-Alikes. 9: (3-4) Oct., 1982.
- Pharm Chem Newsletter, The Look-Alikes Explosion. 2: (3) May, June, 1982.
- Siegel, R.K., Cocaine smoking. J. Psychoactive Drugs. 14: 271-343, 1982.

33. Over-the-Counter Medicines: Psychophysiologic Reactions

The proprietary or over-the-counter business is a multibillion-dollar industry that spends 20 to 40 percent of its gross income on advertising. If some visitor from outer space were to learn about us from our television commercials, he, she, or it would have to conclude that we are a seriously infirm race.

We cannot sleep, yet have difficulties staying awake. We sniffle, sneeze, or cough incessantly without the appropriate medicaments. We have an unserviceable digestive tract from stem to stern, indigestion and hemorrhoids being only two of its many afflictions. Our teeth and skins are remarkably untidy, and the odor of the human body is a matter of grave universal concern.

Fortunately, the visitor would learn from television that we have discovered remedies that ameliorate or cure us of what we have or are. Unfortunately, this conclusion is not borne out by OTC drug evaluations of the FDA, which found two-thirds of these nostrums to be "ineffective" or "probably ineffective" and that careful studies have never been done to prove their efficacy. So the worth of the remedies offered to us by some handsome man or beautiful woman who proffers a package of the product, oddly enough, close to their right ear, is very much in doubt.

ADVERSE REACTIONS

When taken in larger than recommended amounts, or when used persistently over many years, some of the OTC medications have a potential for harm. Although they may be no more effective than a placebo, they are not as safe—especially not for the very young, the aged, or the very ill. This essay will deal only with some of the psychophysiologic misfortunes that can occasionally befall the consumer of these almost unregulated, but widely used patent medicines.

189

SCOPOLAMINE PSYCHOSIS

The acute confusional states associated with disorientation, hallucinations, delusions, and attentional difficulties are among the most common of the undesired reactions to a number of proprietary medicines.

The medications used for sleep (Sominex, Sleep-Eze, Compoz, etc.) all contain scopolamine, an atropine-related alkaloid. Anticholinergic toxicity occurs, including dilated, fixed pupils, dry mouth, a flushed dry skin, a rapid pulse, and a florid delirium. Ordinarily, much more than the recommended two tablets must be taken in order to produce the delirium. Such overdosing can occur when the average amount does not procure sleep, when amnesia for having taken the medication intervenes, or when a suicide is attempted.

Alternatively, the patient may already be on one of the many medications with anticholinergic effects for Parkinsonism, gastric distress, depression, or other emotional disorders, and an atropine-like psychosis results from the scopolamine plus the other anticholinergic drug.

Ullman and Groh found that physicians working in a Washington, D.C., emergency room had to differentiate scopolamine psychosis from acute schizophrenia with fair regularity. When the diagnosis turned out to be a toxic psychosis due to scopolamine, it was confirmed by thin layer chromatography for methapyrilene and salicylamide, also present in OTC sleep aids, since only one percent of scopolamine is excreted in the urine. However, even so small an amount will dilate a cat's eye if a drop of urine containing scopolamine is instilled. The hypodermic injection of 10 to 30 mg of methacholine, a cholinergic drug, will produce flushing, sweating, salivation, lacrimation, and intestinal hyperactivity if an anticholinergic like scopolamine is *not* present.

The treatment should also establish the diagnosis. One or two injections of 2 mg of physostigmine intramuscularly or intravenously will produce rapid clearing of the sensorium if scopolamine or another anticholinergic drug is the cause of the delirium, especially if the intoxication has been recent. Since physostigmine is short-acting, it may require hourly injections in severe instances of poisoning. Diazepam will help control combativeness and should prevent convulsions.

SYMPATHOMIMETIC PSYCHOSIS

Infrequently, the overuse of nasal sprays, antiasthmatics, weight-reducing agents, or cough and cold preparations induces an amphetamine-like psychosis. Patent medicines may contain ephedrine, phenylephrine, naphazoline, phenylpropanolamine, or other mild stimulants. Although mild, enormous quantities may be used. As an example, the swelling of the mucous membranes of the nose may be briefly reduced following some spray or nose drop instillation containing one of the sympathomimetic drugs. A reactive hyperemia of the membranes, however, will promptly occlude the nasal passages requiring more of the same treatment for relief. Snow et al. reported one person who used a phenylephrine nasal spray every 15 minutes while awake for 13 years, culminating in a toxic psychosis.

Both ephedrine and phenylpropanolamine are appearing in laboratory reports of street drug analyses. They are being used as adulterants for amphetamine and cocaine. Although less stimulating than the amphetamines, if a sufficient quantity is swallowed, an equivalent psychostimulation is possible. These drugs appear in cold, cough, and asthma preparations.

In addition, phenylpropanolamine can be found in large doses in the OTC antiobesity agents. The OTC weight reducers are a highly advertised and briskly expanding market. It is predictable that phenylpropanolamine will be used more frequently for its euphoric effects and as an adulterant for stimulants like amphetamine and cocaine. People with high blood pressure should take such medications only under supervision.

Naturally, the paraphernalia shops are in the act, too. They are selling "Pseudocaine," "Coco Snow," "Real Caine," and "Rock Crystal," usually combinations of ephedrine, phenylpropanolamine, and procaine as a sort of poor man's cocaine. Apparently, this is not illegal in many states.

BROMISM

Although bromism has decreased considerably in the past quarter century, it has not disappeared. A diminishing number of OTC formulations contain bromide salts. Chronic bromism is manifested by a toxic psychosis, a rash that is usually acneform, and cerebellar signs. Bromide levels above 9 mEq/liter are indicative of bromide poisoning.

SALICYLISM

The high-dose, chronic use of salicylates (aspirin, salicylamide) can induce a toxic psychosis not too different from that observed with chronic bromism. In addition to the delirium and the skin and cerebellar changes, a metabolic acidosis resulting in hyperventilation and tinnitus with hearing loss may be present. Analgesic nephropathy is another cause of concern. Although the phenacetin in preparations like APC was considered the cause of the papillary renal necrosis, it is now believed that massive amounts of salicylates contribute to this kidney disorder.

Bleeding from the stomach might occur even at average doses of aspirin. It is due to a direct erosive effect upon the gastric lining and a lowering of the prothrombin level. Acute salicylate poisoning is one of the more common causes of accidental death due to chemicals. Children may succumb to the accidental swallowing of as little as 10 grams of aspirin (15–650 mg tablets).

TYLENOL TOXICITY

If, by substituting acetaminophen (Tylenol, Vanquish, etc.) we assumed that we were avoiding the problems with salicylates, the emerging facts do not seem to bear it out. The advertising just has not caught up with the facts. When higher than the recommended doses are taken, liver necrosis, a serious to fatal complication, can occur. Heavy users of alcohol and aminoacetophen are particularly vulnerable to severe liver damage. As with aspirin and other salicylates, acute kidney necrosis can develop from prolonged high dosage use, a not too uncommon situation in searchers after relief from pain. So all minor analgesics are unsafe when misused.

DEPENDENCE

Dependency states in connection with the compulsive ingestion of sleep aids, bromides, and minor analgesics like aspirin and phenacetin are infrequent, but they are known to occur. These substances provide poor quality "highs" and drunken states. Proprietary medicines containing sympathomimetics (Dristan, Contac, etc.) in their formulation are more frequently abused for their euphoriant effect. The following two substances, codeine and the antihistamines, also are capable of producing dependency states.

CODEINE

The overuse of codeine-containing cough mixtures (terpin hydrate with codeine, Cheracol with codeine, etc.) is by no means rare. In the most recent high school senior survey, 10 percent reported that they have used opiates other than heroin at least one time not under a doctor's prescription. Since codeine cough syrup is the easiest opiate to obtain, it may be assumed that this substance was the item used in most instances. Heroin addicts who cannot "score" and polydrug users drink codeine cough syrups by the bottle.

The codeine cough syrups contain 10mg/5ml or 60 mg/ounce of codeine. They are usually sold in four-ounce bottles that contain 240 mg of codeine. In the case of the elixir of terpin hydrate with codeine, its alcohol content is equivalent to that of 80-proof bourbon, so this adds to its popularity. It has become such a problem that it cannot be purchased without a prescription in some states. Empty codeine cough syrup bottles can be seen scattered over the streets near pharmacies where they can be bought without a prescription.

Just why codeine cough syrups have been kept on the OTC market is difficult to understand. A four-ounce bottle of cough syrup provides the equivalent of 20 to 25 mg of oral morphine and can initiate or support an opiate type of dependence. If cough suppression is desired, it can be achieved just as well with dextromethorphan as with codeine. The former drug is not dependency producing nor does it have analgesic effects. It also does not induce drowsiness or constipation.

ANTIHISTAMINES

The antihistamines pervade the over-the-counter market. They appear in cold remedies, cough syrups, sleeping potions, allergy preparations, antimotion sickness relievers, and analgesics. The major problem associated with their use is undesired somnolence. Although this effect is exploited when it is included in the sleep aids, many of the other indications require daytime administration, and the sedation becomes a burden that can be dangerous when operating a car, airplane, or heavy machinery.

The antihistamines are sometimes sought out by those who want a barbiturate type of "high." In large amounts they can provide an intoxicated state resembling the barbiturate hypnosedatives except for the fixed, dilated pupils that accompany antihistamine poisoning.

SUMMARY

For benign, self-limiting conditions there is no reason why OTC preparations should not be available. If symptom relief from nonthreatening conditions is desired, self-medication with safe preparations is not objectionable. However, not all the medicines available for purchase at drug stores and supermarkets are effective or completely safe and when used in large amounts or for extended periods some can be hazardous.

BIBLIOGRAPHY

- Hall, R.C. et al. Psychiatric and physiological reactions produced by over-the-counter medications. *J. Psychedelic Drugs*. 10:243–249, 1978.
- Medical Letter. Over-the-counter cough remedies, 21:103–104, 1979.

- Murray, R.M. Minor analgesic abuse: The slow recognition of a public health problem. *Brit. J. Addic.* 75:9–17, 1980.
- Snow, S.S., Logan, T.P. and Hollender, M.H. Nasal spray addiction and psychosis: A case report. *Brit. J. Psychiat.* 136:297–299, 1980.
- Ullman, K.C. and Groh, R.H. Identification and treatment of acute psychotic states secondary to the usage of over-the-counter sleeping preparations. *Amer. J. Psychiat.* 128:1244–1248, 1972.

34. The Hallucinogens

Hallucinogens are among the most ancient drugs, but it was LSD (d-lysergic acid diethylamide) that ushered in the current wave of nonmedical drug use a quarter century ago. Since those heady days, its popularity has waxed and waned. Recent reports indicate that a resurgence of LSD usage is under way. The common, typical hallucinogens include LSD, mescaline, and psilocybin, but hundreds of others are known.

THE NATURE OF THE STATE

The reason for these drugs' attractiveness must be grasped to understand the popularity of the psychotomimetic series. In amounts noted in Table 34-1 or larger, these substances produce dose-related changes in perception, thinking, emotion, arousal, and self-image that are unusual during sober consciousness. Autonomic signs are few, the most obvious being pupilary dilation.

An inhibition in the dampening of sensory input produces a flood of sensation. Colors and sounds are more intense. Subjective time is slowed. Synesthesias, the overflow of one sensory mode into another, are often described. What is perceived takes on an intensified significance. Illusions are common as are pseudohallucinations (a misperception that is recognized as a misperception), but true hallucinations are actually infrequent despite the name given to the class.

The cognitive alterations include a decrease in logical thought with increased eidetic imagery. What is thought is visualized. "Knight's move" thinking is described with jumps over logical sequences and with nonlinear conclusions that appear to the user to be more valid than ordinary thought processing. At higher doses, cognition seems to fuse with percepts and feelings into a primordial thinking-feeling-sensing pattern. A paranoid thought distortion is often encountered in which the individual has megalomaniacal notions of omnipotence and less frequently, delusions of suspicion and persecution.

The emotional response to an hallucinogen can vary from an ecstatic, bliss-

Table 34–1
Classification of the Major Hallucinogenic Drugs

	Derived From	Average Dose (Oral)	Popular Street Name
I. Those with an indole nucleus			
LSD	Ergot fungus	0.1 mg	Acid
Psilocybin	Psilocybe mushroom	10 mg	Mushrooms
DMT	Cohaba snuff, synthetic	50 mg, smoked	
II. Those with a phenethylamine nucleus			
Mescaline	Peyote cactus	400 mg	Mesc
DOM	Amphetamine derivative	4 mg	STP
MDA	Amphetamine derivative	100 mg	
III. Atypical hallucinogens			
PCP (phencyclidine)	Synthetic	5 mg	Angel dust, etc.
Ketamine	Synthetic	500 mg, I.M.	Green
THC	Cannabis	30 mg	Pot, hash

ful, contentless feeling to a miserable, hopeless dysphoria. The former is called the chemical transcendental state, the latter is the "bummer," a panicky belief that one is insane or mentally fragmented and will remain so. By far, the most common reason for taking psychedelic drugs is the expectation of a "high," euphoria.

The changes in self-image are substantial. The ego boundaries loosen and dissolve. This results either in a sense of oneness and fusion with the universe or feelings of being inextricably lost. The observer self is attenuated, accounting for the ideas of enhanced creativity and even omniscience. Depersonalization and derealization produce either an ego syntonic state of oneness with everyone and everything, or the opposite, a feeling of complete isolation.

Hallucinogens can be profoundly attractive as euphoriants, or to those who seek a chemically induced transcendent experience. The state can also be profoundly disruptive. Serious temporary or long-lasting decompensations will be described.

THE ATYPICAL HALLUCINOGENS

The indoleamine and the phenethylamine hallucinogens can produce the mental changes noted above. The atypical hallucinogens evoke similar changes, but have additional effects that differentiate them. In addition, while cross tolerance to LSD, mescaline, and psilocybin has been demonstrated, cross tolerance to the atypical hallucinogens does not occur.

Phencyclidine (PCP) and Ketamine

These hallucinogens are representative of a series of arylcyclohexamines that have numerous neurologic and autonomic manifestations. The neurologic signs include lateral and vertical nystagmus, gait ataxia, dysarthria, muscle rigidity, major convulsions, and an eyes-open coma when large amounts are taken. The analgesia and unconsciousness have prompted their use as dissociative anesthetics. The autonomic findings include hypertension, tachycardia, sweating, flushing, and gastrointestinal atony.

Complicated alterations of mentation and neurologic, autonomic, and behavioral functions occur because the PCP analogues affect all neurotransmitter systems, particularly the catecholaminergic, serotonergic, cholinergic, and anticholinergic neuronal functions. A specific PCP receptor site on certain neurons has been postulated.

THC

THC, the active principle in *cannabis sativa*, is a water-insoluble, lipid-soluble cannabinoid that accounts for most of the psychic and somatic effects of smoking marijuana or hashish. The low-dose state is a relaxed, dreamy reverie. Larger amounts induce illusions, pseudohallucinations, and paranoid thought alterations. In addition, autonomic effects include tachycardia and vasodilation such as conjunctival injection (red eye), hypothermia, and postural hypotension.

Other drugs

Other drug classes can induce the phenomena described under "The Nature of the State." These include anticholinergics, the withdrawal syndromes of alcohol and other central nervous depressants, opiates, certain anesthetics, and other chemicals that distort cerebral metabolism. These tend to resemble deliria with confusion and disorientation as presenting symptoms. The mental alterations induced by amphetamines and cocaine are more difficult to differentiate from the hallucinogenic experience.

DIAGNOSIS

The uncomplicated hallucinogenic experience rarely comes to the attention of the physician. It is the untoward effects that bring the user to the attention of the health care professional. Acute anxiety, panic, and psychotic episodes can occur, and these require precise identification. Often the history of recent consumption of the hallucinogen is provided by the patients or those who accompany them. Urine or blood screens are worth taking because the alleged drug may have been adulterated with another agent. THC and PCP are identifiable by commercial laboratories, but LSD cannot be tested for except in research laboratories that have interest in the latter drug.The anxiety and panic states tend to be transient, clearing within a day or two. More prolonged psychotic depressions and anxiety reactions occur. These represent the disrupting effect of the negative psychedelic experience upon psychological homeostasis, or the precipitation of an underlying, latent disorder by the stress of the hallucinogenic experience. For example, the upsurge of repressed material under LSD can induce a prolonged schizophrenic or briefer schizophreniform reaction. Organic brain damage has not been conclusively proven to occur in connection with the typical hallucinogens. The flashback is a syndrome idiosyncratic to the psychotomimetic agents. It represents a recurrence of some aspect of the hallucinogenic experience days or months after consuming these drugs. Ordinarily, flashbacks disappear with time and reassurance, but they can be upsetting, emerging as they do without a perceptible cause. These recrudescences are not due to a retention of the drug. LSD, for example, has a half-life of three hours.

The diagnosis of a PCP reaction requires additional comment. The PCP psychosis resembles acute paranoid schizophrenia even more than symptoms caused by the typical hallucinogens. During the early period of PCP overuse, many patients were admitted to hospitals with a diagnosis of acute paranoid schizophrenia. It was only during the weeks of recovery that the history of phencyclidine consumption was elicited. It is worthwhile to do urine testing for PCP, amphetamines, and cocaine in all patients with acute psychotic reactions.

The combination of an acute or subacute psychotic or depressive state with the neurologic and autonomic changes mentioned above is diagnostic of phencyclidine psychosis. Unpredictable, belligerent behavior also seems to accompany PCP use more than with the other hallucinogens. Reports of extraordinary strength are frequent, and they also characterize the phencyclidine state. Presumably, this can be due to the analgesia and the intense emotional quality of some experiences.

Death due to the typical hallucinogens is most infrequent. Chronic organ toxicity is unknown. When death occurs, it is in connection with the drug-induced mental aberrations. Accidental death is the most often encountered, caused by serious misinterpretations of the environment or of oneself. For example, people have drowned or sustained fatal falls apparently while under the impression they could walk on water or fly. Suicides have occurred during the posthallucinogen state from depression or fears of remaining psychotic. Very few homicides have been reported. These have tended to be bizarre in nature, often involving repetitive stabbings without particular motives.

TREATMENT

Most hallucinogenic experiences never achieve medical visibility. Of those that do, support, reassurance, and a quiet environment in the company of a family or staff member with whom the patient is comfortable are usually sufficient to reduce the dysphoria. Overdose of drugs like LSD and mescaline are essentially unknown. Ordinarily, after a night's observation and sleep, the emergency is resolved. A sedative may be used because the hallucinogenic state is one of hyperalertness. Suggestion is a potential therapeutic aid, but the hypersuggestibility of the patient may also result in increasingly disturbed reactions if the paranoid nature of the thought process is not appreciated. Prolonged psychoses require neuroleptics. Whether or not consistent use of hallucinogens produces organic brain damage is not proven, although such usage can lead to attenuation of appropriate social behaviors. Consistent phencyclidine use is reported to be associated with neuropsychological deficits.

The management of phencyclidine toxicity is substantially different. Overdose is a possibility and requires diligent intervention. Since PCP is acidophillic, urinary acidification and continuous gastric suction accelerate its excretion. The hypertension may require treatment to prevent cerebral hemorrhage. Prophylactic diazepam or high-dose phenytoin should be considered to avoid convulsions. Five-point restraints may be required for excessive hyperactivity. In some instances the muscular activity is so extreme that myoglobinuria with tubular necrosis is a possibility. Tracheal intubation may be needed and should be done by an experienced anesthesiologist because laryngospasm is readily induced. Drugs for the psychotic reactions are the neuroleptics; chlorpromazine and haloperidol are the most frequently used.

The management of flashbacks often requires nothing more than providing information about its cause and its generally favorable prognosis. Flashbacks are sometimes precipitated by stress, antihistamines, marijuana, and fatigue. These should be avoided when a flashback has occurred. It would be unusual to experience a flashback after a year has passed without one.

SUMMARY

The hallucinogens are a group of drugs that are attractive for a variety of reasons. Their popularity has waxed and waned over time, and there is no reason to believe that they will disappear. The chemical visionary state attracts some; more look for euphoria and sensory intensification from these agents. The paradox is that although they are mysticomimetic, they are also psychotomimetic. The higher risk drugs, like phencyclidine, deserve a permanent disappearance; the risk-benefit ratio for the user is much too narrow.

It is the management of dysfunctional behavior that is most important. Prolonged psychoses and panic states are less common and persistent physiological disturbances are rare.

V
HOW DRUGS
CHANGE PEOPLE
AND SOCIETY

35. Coming of Age
in America—with Drugs:
Contemporary Adolescence

It is becoming clear that a drug-free Eden, if it ever existed, will never return. The days when youth had no access or interest in the bewildering array of consciousness-transforming drugs will, in all likelihood, not be seen again. We can expect ebbs and surges of psychochemical usage for what is called "recreation," but a return to an era when adolescent drug abuse did not exist is difficult to visualize.

This is so for two reasons. For one, it seems impossible to interdict more than a fraction of the traffic, and the supply side of the equation is an important contributory factor. Where drugs are available and affordable, some people will use them. The second reason is the changes in social structure and in the growing-up processes that have taken place in the past half century. Relaxed societal taboos against the nonmedical use of drugs, and the fact that decisions about using drugs are being made by juveniles, make a reversal of these trends problematic. At what age is a youngster capable of making decisions about drugs—decisions that can impact on his or her health and future? The obvious answer is: when mature decisions can be made, and when sufficient accurate information about the drug is acquired. Unfortunately, it seems that an inverse relationship exists between maturity and information when they are correlated with dangerous drug usage.

So for a while, we can expect a situation in which a smorgasbord of psychoactive drugs is available, and young people will taste them. On the latter point, the figures are impressive. The number of 18- to 25-year-olds who had ever tried marijuana rose from 4 percent in 1962 to 68 percent in 1980. Those in the same age group who had ever tried illicit drugs other than marijuana went from 3 percent to 33 percent during the same time interval. These data are scary, but on reflection, not really meaningful. So what if a majority of young adults have "ever used" some illicit drug? We know that adolescence is a period of exploratory, risk-taking, sensation-seeking behavior, and now chemical exploration is a part of that world. What is much more significant is: how many go on to use drugs dysfunctionally? This number is more difficult to obtain, because it includes not only the heavy user of any drug that is intoxicating, but also the one-time user who happens to take too much, or the one who happens to drive a car ineptly while under the influence.

THE CORE ISSUE

The issue really is: how can one come of age in America without becoming a casualty of the acute or chronic use of drugs that affect mood, thinking, and sensing in the process? Admitting that these mind-altering agents will be around, and that many will try them, what can be done to keep the morbidity and mortality down?

The general answer to the question is that those forces that influence adolescent thinking and behavior must be influenced to encourage a nondrug or a nondysfunctional drug existence. The major forces involved can be listed, not in order of their greatest impact for this varies with the young person involved:

1. The family

2. The peers

3. The teachers

4. The electronic media

5. Entertainment and sports figures

6. Religion

Overall, each of these forces have not been too successful in providing positive, life-enhancing, drug-deterring guidance. In fact, some of these forces have had negative consequences insofar as drug usage is concerned.

Efforts to modify the influence of each of the six elements upon youthful development have been attempted. Family action groups for prevention and early intervention have been expanding and offer promising results. Family therapy for young drug users requiring treatment is an important approach. Instead of the usual peer pressures to indulge in drugs positive peer influence groups have been developed that involve either group interaction, information, assistance, or working together in community projects.* Concerned schools and educators have attempted to provide information, a limited amount of counseling, and an environment that discourages drug use.

Since adolescents watch television for more hours than they attend school, television is a potent force in developing attitudes and values. Although occasional exceptions exist, the general tone of television programs tends to represent drug and excessive alcohol use as acceptable or even approving evidence that one is an adult. Many programs and commercials can be cited that support the use of drugs, licit and illicit. While most adults come to develop a doubtful attitude toward both the commercials and the content between the commercials, children and adolescents are more impressionable and less discerning. They receive repetitious covert and overt messages that are less than helpful, and that in fact make using drugs seem normal and acceptable. Not infrequently, adolescents use entertainment and sports figures as models of behavior. Positive messages from these prestigious people contribute to their final attitude toward drug use. On the other hand much of the popular music contains inane or seductive mentions of drug use that tend to move impressionable young people into the drug scene.

The formal religions and the religious equivalents like AA, NA (Narcotics Anonymous), and Synanon have the capability to prevent the involvement of young people in drugs, or of rehabilitating the substance abuser. This may point to a basic need of certain dysfunctional drug abusers—the need to believe in something out there. The lack of a cosmology or belief in the meaningfulness of the universe can be reflected in drug-seeking and other deviant behaviors. A lack of faith in oneself and in existence may be basic to many of what we call "causes" of substance abuse. These would include depression, anxiety, hopelessness, poor self-esteem, directionlessness, and inability to trust. To parahrase the Marxist slogan that "religion is the opium of the people," it may be that "opium is the religion of the unbelieving people." Some sort of an ethic and creed is incorporated in many drug treatment programs, and therapeutic communities, AA, transcendental meditation, and Narconon are only the first examples that come to mind.

It is interesting that certain drugs have sometimes been used to induce a sort of transcendental state—primarily, but not exclusively, the hallucinogens. In one of the sustaining errors in the scientific literature, William James in his *Principles of Psychology* (1907) wrote: "It is the power of alcohol to stimulate the mystical consciousness that has made it such an important substance in Man's history."

---

*These programs are described in Adolescent Peer Pressure: Theory, Correlates and Program Implications for Drug Abuse Prevention, N.I.D.A., D.H.H.S. Publication No. (ADM) 81-1152, U.S. Gov't. Printing Office, Washington, D.C. 20402.

ADOLESCENT ACCESS TO DRUGS

It was rare in many cultures, until recently, to grow up with access to mind-altering agents. It was only at a time of transition from youth into manhood that some deliriant might be used as a rite of passage. Administered as part of an elaborate ritual, a potion like caapi was given to the youthful aspirant before the Yurupari whipping ceremony by some Colombian Indian tribes. In tropical Africa a decoction of the calabar bean (the ordeal bean) was used as a test of readiness for manhood. It is true that adolescent Andean Indians are given coca leaves to chew, but that is only when they start working in the oxygen-poor atmosphere of the Altiplano. Chewing coca leaves under those conditions is hardly a psychostimulant. It serves more as a hunger suppressant and antifatigue potion.

Alcoholic beverages and solvents like gasoline were the intoxicants available to the young. Very few underage people could afford drugs, and if they could, stricter parenting practices than now prevail would not permit it.

That affluent juveniles in the Western world can afford marijuana at $100.00 an ounce, methaqualone at $5.00 a tablet, and even cocaine, is a remarkable, new phenomenon. It means that for the first time, the curiosity and mimicking propensities of young humans can extend to the chemical mood changers. We have some evidence that young people do not handle psychochemicals as well as adults. Part of the reason is that they lack the adaptive mechanisms that must be learned to manage psychological turbulence. Another possibility is that some of the drug-metabolizing enzyme systems are immature. One thing is certain. The earlier a drug habit starts, the more unfavorable the long-term outlook.

Growing up safely and soberly in America is not simple. In some neighborhoods it is deviant to not use drugs. Even rural youth, at one time protected by space and opportunity from urban and suburban drug use patterns, are now involved.

It will take changes over many generations or a revolution of values, child-rearing practices, and morality to definitively alter our current situation. But what can be done now while awaiting gradual or abrupt changes? It seems necessary for each person to assume responsibility for his or her own behaviors, including drug-using behaviors. Parents must begin early to set reasonable limits and give appropriate responsibilities to their children. A return to the ancient Greek idea of a healthy mind in a healthy body would be worth resurrecting. Something to believe in—some faith or system of beliefs—would make life more livable and make drug taking irrelevant.

SUMMARY

The adolescent hazards of the past, starvation, pestilence, and poverty, have given way to the modern plagues of youth, accidents, suicides, and homicides. The interaction of drugs and alcohol with these three current disasters is obvious. The common denominators are the degree of freedom, the lack of responsibility, and the failure of faith that adolescents cannot handle or endure.

Coming of age in America before the present era was far from ideal or idyllic. No one would want to go back to the child labor practices of those "good old days." But something has gone wrong. In the effort to make things better for our children we have succeeded only in making them easier, and that may not be better.

BIBLIOGRAPHY

- Cretcher, D. *Steering Clear: Healing Your Child Through the High Risk Years*. Winston Press, Minneapolis, 1982.
- Henden, H. et al. *Adolescent Marijuana Abusers and Their Families*. NIDA Research Monograph 40. U.S. Government Printing Office, Washington, D.C. 20402, 1981.
- Manatt, M. *Parents, Peers and Pot*. DHEW Publication No. (ADM) 79-812, National Institute on Drug Abuse, Rockville, MD, 1979.
- Resnick, H. and Adams, T. *Channel One: A Government and Private Sector Partnership for Drug Abuse Prevention*. DHHS Publication No. (ADM) 81-1174, U.S. Government Printing Office, Washington, D.C. 20402.

36. Drug Abuse: Predisposition and Vulnerability

The only drug for which a genetic predisposition has substantial scientific support is alcohol. The twin studies done in Scandinavia and the United States convince most investigators that certain alcoholics possess a trait that makes them more susceptible to overdrinking. Whether this is a psychological or a physiological burden is unclear.

Claims that opiate dependence is a metabolic disease have been made by Dole and Nyswander on the basis of the "consistent therapeutic response of previously intractable addicts to adequate doses of methadone. The biologic expression of the disease is an abnormal appetite for the narcotic drugs." Now that endogenous opioids and narcotic receptor sites have been identified, the concept has been brought up to date by postulating a deficiency in endogenous opioid functioning. While hypoendorphinism or hypoenkephalism may, one day, be identifiable disorders, much more research will have to be done before opiate dependence is shown to have a primary metabolic etiology. The first question that comes to mind in attempting to ascribe intrinsic metabolic deficiencies to heroinism is: Why have so many addicts succeeded in overcoming the disorder without opiate maintenance? The second question is: Why have many failed in trials of opiate maintenance? Many other questions remain.

Very recently an assumption was made that cocaine dependence was caused by a catecholaminergic deficiency on the basis of three cases having been improved with methylphenidate (Ritalin) maintenance. Such speculations are interesting, but not convincing. To my knowledge no other drug or drug class has been claimed to have a biologic substrate. In view of the increasing polydrug pattern of abuse and the shifting of drug habits from narcotics to central nervous depressants to hallucinogens to stimulants, in random sequence, it is just as well.

Psychological predispositions exist, as can be noted in epidemiologic studies. Schizophrenics, borderline personalities, depressives, and antisocial personalities are overrepresented in such surveys. Insofar as sociopathy is

208

concerned, we must be cautious about making the diagnosis hastily in drug-dependent people. Their life style demands sociopathic behavior. I have been impressed at how the antisocial manifestations disappear following successful treatment. Aphoric people, those who are unable to feel deeply, are also likely to find relief from their distressing symptoms with psychochemicals.

When I go into a neighborhood in south central Los Angeles and learn that most of the young males are on heroin or other drugs, I wonder why the small minority is not. Surely they have been exposed. A certain amount of peer pressure must have been exerted. Why did they resist?

Factors listed below contribute to the vulnerability to abused substances. Studying their opposites might tell us why certain people remain uninvolved.

LOW THRESHOLDS FOR AMBIGUITY, DISSONANCE, AND FRUSTRATION; OR HIGH LEVELS OF ANXIETY, HOPELESSNESS AND HELPLESSNESS

Those people with chronically noxious feelings and the inability to cope with those feelings obtain so much relief from drugs that they are to be found in higher percentages among the dysfunctional users of any intoxicant. They seek the feelings of power and competence that amphetamines and cocaine bring, the distancing from cares that opiates achieve, or the relaxation of tensions that accompanies the depressant drugs. For people in distress, the drug experience produces a euphoric interlude far greater than for the rest of us.

AVAILABILITY

Low cost and easy availability of mind-changing drugs are obvious elements that favor widespread, inordinate consumption in any population. We are witnessing this now in urban cities of Peru with coca paste, in metropolitan Bangkok with heroin, and, until recently, in Southern California with phencyclidine. High cost and the fear of buying poor-quality material do not necessarily bar excessive use, as we see in the spreading cocaine craze.

FRIENDSHIP GROUP PRESSURES

Much drug experimentation and abuse starts at an age when peers and older siblings exert greater impact on the shaping of behavior than do parents. The group leader is an especially potent molder of attitudes and values. It is within the friendship group that learning how and what to inhale, smoke, shoot, or score occurs.

ROLE MODELING

When adults close to the individual or when admired figures in sports, entertainment, or other prominent activities demonstrate that drug taking is approved or even acceptable, the mimicking predisposition of adolescents invites imitation.

POVERTY AND AFFLUENCE

Although the lifestyle that accompanies poverty can induce a negative emotional state that drives one toward drug abuse, so can affluence. Under both conditions, the young tend to lose their goals and their way. Superficially, it would seem that being poor might offer some protection against the overuse of drugs. But this is not so—the highest priority is given to the purchase of drugs. Being affluent makes a drug career a readily available option without the deterrent effect of having to find money for it. The penetration of drug dependence into the middle class is one noteworthy aspect of the current drug scene.

THE FAMILY

It is almost trite to say that the disrupted family can play a role in the move toward dysfunctional drug use. Family turmoil is a heavy load for children to bear. But the intact, loving family is no guarantee of nonusage by the offspring; other factors may be too overwhelming.

EUPHORIA AND DYSPHORIA

The rewarding aspects of drug use, especially at the outset, provide positive conditioning to continue the pursuit of pleasure through chemicals. When life becomes tougher because of chronic drug use, or when efforts are made to stop the practice, the dysphoria leads to negative conditioning and perpetuates drug use. It might be imagined that the loss of health, family, job, self-esteem, and the other punishments that come with the consistent overuse of drugs will lead to cessation. It is not quite so. Instead, this misery can lead to continued use.

CURIOSITY

Curiosity, the willingness to take a drug once or twice, does not sustain long-term use. The "ever-used" statistic that epidemiologists collect has no public health significance.

CRAVING

Craving has no meaning to someone who has never used drugs, but it is a potent force in keeping a person on the usage escalator. It consists, in addition to the conditionings already mentioned, of the nondrug reinforcing properties of consistent use. The stimuli of the presence of the drug, the people with whom one has fixed, and other stimuli of the rewarding event all become positive reinforcers, sometimes intensely so. Craving occurs a few hours after last use, during withdrawal, and for weeks or months after abstinence has begun.

THE PHARMACOLOGIC IMPERATIVES

Clearly, after physical dependence has developed, the urge to continue using is great, so great that efforts to induce the individual to enter treatment without coercion of some sort are likely to fail. Another mechanism exists that has little to do with physical dependence and makes discontinuance problematic or, if it has somehow been achieved, frequently causes relapse. I am referring to the use of rapid delivery systems to introduce alleged "nonaddicting" drugs into the body, specifically cocaine.

What cocaine does, when injected intravenously or smoked as freebase, is to provide a very high "high" lasting a minute, sometimes two. As brain-cocaine levels decrease the mood returns to baseline. During a cocaine binge the injections or the puffs may be repeated every few minutes. The hyperphoria diminishes over time, and dysphoria is experienced as the effect wears off. Here are two enormously reinforcing events occurring with great frequency and intensity. The third lock that such cocaine use has on the heavy user is the "crash," or withdrawal syndrome, manifested by a considerable depression, probably due to an exhaustion of dopamine and the dopaminergic receptor cells in the reward centers. The depression is briefly "cured" by more cocaine. Finally when intravenous cocaine hydrochloride or smoked cocaine alkaloid are used over months or years, the threshold for experiencing life's ordinary pleasures is elevated. Nothing is enjoyable—except cocaine. So abstinence is a drab, dismal, aphoric existence for many weeks until the exhaustion of the reward system recedes. These are four reasons why persistent cocaine users are vulnerable to continue using or to return to using; only one reason involves physical dependence.

DISCUSSION

The reasons given by the person overinvolved in drugs for his or her vulnerability are sometimes meaningful, but sometimes are rationalizations. It is natural to overemphasize the cause "out there" rather than any inadequacies

212 THE SUBSTANCE ABUSE PROBLEMS: NEW ISSUES

within. This is understandable since we all use the same projections when explaining our own defects. The underlying causes are multifactorial, hardly to be satisfactorily explained by "curiosity" or "my boy friend turned me on" or some similar statement.

The array of predisposing and vulnerable factors presented here is incomplete, but they probably cover most of the more common elements in arriving at a state of destructive drug use. These factors have been present during every epoch, in every land. It becomes necessary to ask why drug abuse is so prevalent in some time and in some places, and not in others.

To me, the major variables are availability and decadence (which is a combination of loss of goals, values, and responsibility on a personal and a national level). To these must be added the freedom to become addicted, for highly repressive political systems are capable of suppressing individual opportunities to overindulge.

And now, to try to answer the question I posed earlier: Why do a few remain abstinent when those around them are altering their mental state with drugs? It seems that some are motivated to avoid drugs through fear, appropriate fear. Some have a vision of the future and want to become somebody. A few might abstain because of parental influences. And there may be one or two who are so deviant that they defy their cultural norms by rebelling and refusing to use.

37. Prescribing Practices: Drug Misuse and Abuse

The abuse of prescription drugs is hardly new. Controlled sedatives, stimulants, and analgesics have been sold on the street alongside hallucinogens, heroin, marijuana, and other illicit drugs. It is not known how much physicians contribute to the diversion of supplies into nonmedical channels, but every effort should be made to keep the amount to a minimum.

Dealers obtain prescription items by warehouse thefts, hijackings, pharmacy burglaries, and collusion with unethical pharmacists and other health care personnel. Theft from physicians and improper prescribing practices add significant amounts to the pool of abusable drugs. The smuggling of drugs and look-alikes from abroad has recently become a major source of supply. At present, methaqualone (Quaalude), either the actual chemical or as tablets made from diazepam, is flooding the market in some cities. Its country of origin seems to be Colombia.

NEW PRESCRIPTION DRUG ABUSES

Two new drug combinations have become popular in recent years: Ts and blues and loads. Ts and blues are Talwin and pyribenzamine. They are consumed, usually orally, in the midwestern cities, but their use is spreading to other parts of the country. Loads were first identified in Los Angeles County. They are a combination of codeine and Doriden. These sedative-narcotic combinations are preferred to the weak heroin that is available.

There is nothing particularly unique about these specific combinations; it is more a matter of availability and fashion. Darvon has been substituted for the Talwin, and any hypnosedative for the Doriden and pyribenzamine.

These latest fads with controlled substances underline the part that medically useful drugs play in the drug abuse problem. The practice is part of a polydrug abuse pattern with alcohol and marijuana almost invariably consumed at the same time. The synergistic effect of these central nervous system depressants makes accidental or intentional overdose a possible outcome.

SPECIAL PROBLEMS IN PRESCRIBING
PSYCHOTROPIC DRUGS

Some guidelines are offered to discourage the misuse and abuse of prescribed drugs.

Leftover Drugs

Stockpiles of mood-altering drugs accumulate in the family medicine cabinet and serve as introductory supplies for youthful members of the family. School surveys report that unused medicines were an important source of initial drug usage among adolescents.

It is undesirable to prescribe an analgesic or hypnotic in amounts exceeding the calculated need. Acute pain (as from a dental extraction) or acute situational insomnia require only a few doses of a drug. Prescribing large amounts is wasteful and can become a part of the hoard of potentially abused drugs.

The Purposeful Patient

People with real or contrived illnesses will visit a series of physicians and clinics to acquire prescriptions for depressants or stimulants for the purpose of becoming intoxicated on the medication. Sorting out malingerers, hypochondriacs, hysterics, and people with difficult to diagnose painful or emotional disorders is one of the more difficult problems in the practice of medicine.

Some of the "con" games patients play include a fictitious history of flank pain and hematuria, genuine abcesses that are not allowed to heal, or well-learned symptoms of chronic relapsing pancreatitis supported by a note from some out-of-town doctor.

It is in the best interest of the patient to refuse to continue to supply some psychotropic drug that he or she had abused. The patient's threat to obtain it from another physician or from the street is no reason to be manipulated into continuing to order the drug.

The "Scrip Doc"

It has been estimated that less than 1 percent of doctors deliberately overprescribe psychotropic drugs for profit. This practice can vary from a prescription mill operation where a "scrip" is written every few minutes for a fee to the gullible physician who acquires the reputation of being an easy mark. Other health care professionals with access to controlled drugs or prescriptions can become a major source of street drugs. Community epidemics of methylphenidate (Ritalin), methaqualone (Quaalude), and propoxyphene (Darvon) abuse flared up after one or a few doctors handed out hundreds of prescriptions. For example, a few years ago a single doctor was responsible for the diversion of 2.5 percent of the national output of Ritalin.

The Unsupervised Patient

Patients given psychotropic drugs without careful periodic review of their status and their total drug consumption from all sources may, intentionally or unintentionally, slip into a pattern of increasing the dose, especially as tolerance develops. Eventually, the physician may be confronted with a patient in distress because the medicine cannot be stopped without inducing withdrawal symptoms.

Defensive Prescribing

It is hardly necessary to mention that before prescribing psychoactive drugs, a history and physical examination should be performed and recorded. The prescription is also recorded in order to provide a numerical basis for supervising the patient's drug usage. Since antianxiety, anti-insomnia, analgesic, and weight-control pharmacotherapy ordinarily represent symptomatic management, additional, concurrent, nondrug methods of dealing with these problems are advisable.

Poor Prescription Security

A pad of prescriptions is priceless to the drug-dependent person. Patients and office workers should not be exposed to the temptation of prescription forms thoughtlessly left lying about. The least that can happen would be a visit from a drug enforcement official asking why thousands of mood elevators or depressants have been ordered for nonexistent patients.

Prescription security can be improved with the following measures:

1. Order prescription blanks that are numbered consecutively so that missing forms can be detected.

2. Use as few pads as possible at any one time.

3. Lock all unused pads in a safe place.

4. Do not sign blanks or put the registration number on in advance.

5. Write prescriptions in ink or indelible pencil.

6. Write for the number of dosage units in such a way that the amount cannot be boosted.

7. Do not use the prescription form as scratch paper. It might be erased and used. Refill information should be filled out, or the patient will do it.

8. Do not throw away obsolete prescription pads. They should be destroyed.

Poor Safeguarding of Supplies

The theft of physicians' bags left in locked cars takes only a minute longer than pilfering from unlocked cars. Repeated office break-ins will occur when a person seeking drugs discovers that entry is easy or learns that large quantities of drugs or needles are routinely stocked.

The Impaired Physician

Impaired physicians, particularly those impaired by drug or alcohol dependence, can become a source of illicit drug supplies. Their own excessive use of psychochemicals may be reflected in an overgenerous prescribing pattern. If their private practice is failing because they can no longer render adequate service, they tend to become "scrip docs" in order to earn a living. This group is also vulnerable to drug blackmail by anyone who knows of their personal problem.

The Counterproductive Third Party Payment System

Certain regulations of third party payers impede good medical practice. For example, chronically anxious or depressed patients or those in continuing pain may be allowed only one visit a month. This requires the prescribing of larger than desirable amounts of psychotropic drugs, which can be abused or employed for purposes of suicide. Under such conditions close supervision is not possible.

COMPLIANCE AND NONCOMPLIANCE

Will a patient take a prescribed drug as ordered? It is estimated that 50 percent of patients deviate from the doctor's directions for using their medication.

The following activities constitute noncompliance on the part of the patients:

1. Never obtaining the prescribed drug.

2. Never taking the prescribed drug.

3. Improper taking of the drug. This may consist of taking it at incorrect intervals, taking incorrect numbers of dosage units a day, omitting dosages, or prematurely discontinuing the drug.

4. Using nonprescribed drugs or taking medication that should have been discontinued. Using alcohol or caffeine along with certain psychotropic drugs adds to or subtracts from their effects.

It is possible to reduce the incidence of noncompliance by increasing the information provided to the patient with the prescription.

1. Inform the patient or the person who will be administering the medication of the reason why the drug is being given.

2. Relate the drug to the condition being treated. If the drug's action will be delayed, as with the tricyclic antidepressants, make this clear. Otherwise the medication may be prematurely abandoned.

3. Provide a precise description, in writing if necessary, of how much, how often, and for how long a time the medication should be used.

4. Indicate what foods, beverages, or other drugs should be avoided while taking the prescribed drug.

5. Explain the more frequent side effects that can occur and what should be done about them (discontinue drugs, call the doctor, etc.). If driving may be impaired, indicate this.

6. Do not make the drug program too complicated. Use as few drugs as infrequently as their pharmacology permits.

7. Review the drug program on each visit. It is sometimes advisable to have the patient bring along all drugs currently used and to count the dosage units when there is suspicion that too much or too little is being used.

8. A drug diary may be helpful in managing certain patients. Every dose of every drug is recorded immediately after ingestion.

9. In other words, prescribing a drug should be regarded as an important procedure.

SUMMARY

At a time when the deliberate chemical alteration of mood states is becoming institutionalized a re-evaluation of our prescribing procedures is warranted. It is true that most of the drugs that arrive at the black marketplace are not medical items and that a substantial proportion of abused prescription drugs are diverted from other points in the supply network. Nevertheless, the amounts deliberately or inadvertently misprescribed by physicians are important in initiating or perpetuating drug abuse. Therefore every effort should be made not to become a part of the drug abuse problem.

38. Substance Abuse: Initiation and Perpetuation

The factors that start someone using drugs for nonmedical purposes are often different from those that produce extended use. Elimination or reduction of the initiating factors constitutes prevention, and treatment is concerned with correction and removal of the applicable perpetuating causes. It is rare that a single cause produces drug-taking behavior, and almost never will persistent drug usage result from one factor alone. As a rule a number of variables interact to determine whether drug experimentation and continued drug misuse will occur.

INITIATING FACTORS

The abusive consumption of drugs usually begins during adolescence or young adulthood, and the very nature of being young contributes to an early involvement with psychochemicals. The elements that encourage drug abuse can be identified as conditions either internal or external to the individual.

Internal Factors

1. Youth is a time of intense exploratory activity, genetically determined for accelerated learning. A "hunger" for new sensations and stimulation will be observed at this time in all species. Curiosity and the search for novel experiences tend to move the young person to explore those altered states of awareness evoked by certain drugs if they are in the environment.

2. Another learning technique is the mimicking behavior of youthful creatures. The adolescent and young adult copies the dress, speech, mannerisms, and, unfortunately, the drug-using patterns of peers. Copying the activities of admired role models such as parents, teachers, friends, and celebrities is an-

219

other way that personal attitudes and desirable or undesirable social behaviors are acquired.

3. Risk taking and incomplete impulse control are characteristic of the young human. These qualities permit drug usage patterns that might be avoided by more mature and cautious individuals. Too many valuable youngsters are lost because of their underdeveloped ability to control their impulses.

4. Young people are more here-and-now oriented and much less concerned with future consequences than older persons. They are also less inclined to delay gratification; in fact, they are disposed to the achievement of pleasure now, including drug-induced euphoria.

5. In present-day North America it is a usual experience for 16- to 25-year-olds to have tried alcohol (95 percent) and marijuana (63 percent) at least once. Therefore, it is easier to look at the nonusing individuals for indicators of their special personality characteristics. The abstainers tend to be more cautious and conforming to established models.

Lifetime use of heroin is much less frequent (3–5 percent), and initial users of this narcotic seem to be more anxious, depressed, frustrated, or antisocial individuals.

External Factors

1. Availability of the substance is, of course, a necessary element. With the recent emergence of stimulant and sedative "look alikes" (ephedrine and phenylpropylamine manufactured to look like one of the amphetamines, and antihistamines made to look like barbiturates or methaqualone), these may become transitional drugs to be used until the real thing becomes accessible.

2. Peer persuasion and peer drug usage are powerful inducements to indulge. It is difficult for someone to abstain over time in the presence of drug-using friends. The desire to identify with and belong and the group's demand for conformity make the use of the group's favorite drug almost inevitable.

3. Familial conflict and disruption will thrust a child toward drug usage, but the converse is not true. Many children from intact, stable, caring families will also try psychochemicals. The quality of a child's upbringing will determine, only in part, whether adolescents will indulge. Peer pressures are more potent instigators of drug experimentation than family influences in many instances.

4. School and social failures tend to encourage drug experimentation. This probably constitutes a search for rewarding experiences that are not available in the course of daily living.

5. The person's societal situation may encourage entry into the drug scene. The wretchedness of some inner city neighborhoods makes escape via drugs almost inevitable. But in a similar fashion, the purposelessness sometimes encountered among juveniles in very affluent neighborhoods can make them high substance abuse areas.

PERPETUATING FACTORS

Although a majority of experimenters will desist from drug use after one or a small number of trials, others continue to indulge. Some will remain occasional consumers. About 10 percent will engage in frequent, heavy use. This latter group tend to be "sicker" emotionally than the nonusers and the "tasters." In fact, their overinvolvement with one or more drugs may be futile efforts at self-treatment of their emotional distress.

A variety of reasons why certain people will continue to imbibe, inhale, inject, or otherwise absorb one or more mind-altering drugs can be identified.

Internal Factors

1. Drugs that induce pleasurable feelings (the "high") or those that lessen unpleasant ones tend to be used repeatedly by people who are unable to enjoy sober consciousness or who suffer from a dysphoric mood state like depression or chronic tension.

2. A sudden feeling of elation (the "rush") is sought after by cocaine, amphetamine, and heroin users. The loss of self, an attenuation or dissolution of the ego boundaries sometimes encountered with the psychedelic drugs, is also repeatedly pursued by certain people.

3. Other rewarding feelings that seem to be relished include intoxication, disinhibition, or stuporousness. These permit a distancing from one's ordinary self or from a miserable reality. Other imagined satisfactions include the defiance of authority and the camaraderie of the common group experience.

4. The rewards may not be as much in the drug taken as in the associated life style. Superficially, it would seem that the strenuous life of the junkie or

of the skid row drunk would have little to commend it. But there are attractions to the street life like casual "friendships" and lack of responsibility. Loneliness is partially overcome, and demanding relationships can be evaded. The "hang loose" street life of the psychedelic ghettos of the 1960s was so attractive that a few of the inhabitants lived the life but did not do drugs.

5. Some of the fun of a drug-using career lies in the fixing. The rituals of repetitively smoking, injecting, or snorting become a part of the reward. The process of preparing a pipe or a marijuana joint becomes a part of a pleasant routine. The tobacco cigarette smoker conditioned by hundreds of puffs a day must find a reward in the mechanics of the busy work of smoking as much as in the taste or the pharmacologic action of the drug.

6. Not pleasure, but the avoidance of withdrawal sickness is an important and frequent reason for continuing to use. Consistent use of sedatives, stimulants, and narcotics induces a distressing withdrawal sickness when they are withheld. The sure knowledge that relief is available from another dose is a powerful inducement to continue the practice.

7. Some drugs, like alcohol in large amounts, are initially associated with pleasure, good cheer, and made-to-order fellowship. In chronic drinkers, however, continued drinking causes a mood shift to anger or depression. The heavy drinker might have an amnesia for the unpleasant period and will recall only the earlier pleasant events. This loss of memory for the negative aspects of the drinking episode encourages further binges.

External Factors

1. The more readily available an abusable substance is, the more likely it is to be used. As specific drugs become more difficult to obtain or more expensive, certain users will reduce or discontinue their habit. Alternatively, they may turn to other psychotropic agents that are less expensive. Consistent users will "stash" or otherwise assure supplies of their intoxicant. Freebase or intravenous cocaine users have difficulty in maintaining a "stash" because of the intense craving to continue use or to obtain relief from a postcocaine depression. When one's favorite drug is inaccessible, a shift to a related drug will take place. When heroin is scarce, codeine cough syrup sales increase.

2. The labelling of a person as an addict is supposed to perpetuate the addict role, according to sociological theory. While labelling may continue the career of an addict in certain instances, it does not appear to be a strong factor in its perpetuation. On the contrary, bringing the person's alcoholism or drug

dependence clearly to awareness may help in achieving the necessary motivation to do something about it.

3. Some drugs, alcohol is the prototype, cause gradual mental impairment to the point where the ability to appreciate the severity of the condition and the ominous outlook if use continues, are lost. In addition, the ability to partially control the use may be eradicated. Under such conditions it is not possible to enlist the patient's cooperation in his or her recovery, and the prognosis becomes much worse.

4. The pharmacology of the drug may be decisive in continued use. Drug-dependent people may become locked into their drug if the withdrawal symptoms or the postdrug depressions are too severe to endure. And others prefer a diminished level of consciousness to their sober, waking awareness.

5. Poor physician management of patients with chronic pain or tension can produce an undesired prolonged dependence on narcotics or sedatives.

SUMMARY

Distinguishing between initiating and perpetuating factors, especially in adolescent drug use, is important. Exploratory drug use may not be associated with social or psychological deviance. The compulsive, continuing consumption of mind-altering drugs is likely to reflect an intrinsic inadequacy in the user and be associated with adverse psychophysical consequences over time. Only a fraction of those who start will continue to use substances dysfunctionally, and as a rule, they are psychologically "sicker." In addition, there are drugs, cocaine, for example, that can overinvolve the most stable and mature among us, given unlimited access.

39. Drugs in the Workplace

Although every type of drug, including heroin and PCP, has been bought, sold, and used during working hours, the principal industrial drugs of concern are alcohol, marijuana, and cocaine. The magnitude of this problem is unquestionable, although it is occasionally denied or ignored.

The Firestone Tire & Rubber Company has completed a study which suggests that drug users were 3.6 times as likely to be involved in a plant accident and were 2.5 times more likely to require absences lasting more than a week than employees who didn't use drugs. Drug users were 5 times as likely to file a workers' compensation claim, and they received 3 times the average level of sick benefits. In addition, they were repeatedly involved in grievance procedures. It was estimated that they functioned at about 67 percent of their work potential. No estimates were made about other damaging aspects of drug abuse at the work site such as thefts of company or other employees' property or funds, or breakage and other kinds of damage to products or equipment.

The Firestone study results are probably representative of industry in general. The human and productivity costs are evidently enormous. Some people believe that the decline in American workers' efficiency and productivity stems from the minority who work under the influence. It is more likely that intoxication during the hours of employment is only one of a number of factors.

ALCOHOL

Alcohol use prior to and during the work day is widespread. Alcohol is consumed in amounts sufficient to impair effectiveness by blue collar, white

---

The material in this chapter was largely derived from three papers presented at a conference on Drugs in Industry, 1982, sponsored by the American Council for Drug Education, Rockville, MD. The papers were: Effects of Marijuana on Skills Performance and Accident Probability, H. Moskowitz, Los Angeles; Marijuana in the Workplace: Mental Effects, S. Cohen, Los Angeles; and, Drug Detection in Industry: Legal Issues, R.T. Angarola, Washington, D.C.

collar, and executive types. Many skills begin to decline at blood levels as low as 0.05 percent. This means that two drinks consumed within an hour on an empty stomach can induce impairment for complex work activities. The 0.05 percent blood level is considered intoxication for purposes of driving a vehicle in some European countries. The industrial accidents, the disabilities, and the breakdowns in interpersonal relationships caused by alcohol excess are so well known that they need no retelling here. Most of the employee assistance programs that many corporations have found valuable for a variety of employee problems were started to deal with problem drinking. For a discussion of occupational alcoholism matters, see: Godwin, D.S. Issues of the Day. *Labor-Management Alcohol Journal* 3:211–213, 1979.

COCAINE

Cocaine is being increasingly used during the workday both for its euphoric effect and for occupational reasons. The latter is an interesting phenomenon that requires additional comment. Professional athletes, entertainment personalities, and business executives may feel unsure of their ability to perform well in their sober state. Before periods of considerable demand on their talents, some will snort cocaine. They seek the overalertness, hypervigilance, speeded-up thoughts, and feeling of competency that small amounts of the drug can provide. Even these amounts, though, can skew the fine tuning of judgment and intricate decision making.

A problem emerges when cocaine is regularly snorted in anticipation of stressful encounters. What happens if cocaine is not at hand and difficult situations arise? Will the absence of one's chemical prosthesis result in subnormal performance? Cocaine is so brief in its action that frequent refills are needed. If they are not at hand, decreasing brain cocaine levels are not conducive to performing at one's optimum.

MARIJUANA

Considerably more information is now available on marijuana's effect on mental functioning, skill performance, and accident probability. Much of these data have not been generally disseminated to the health care professionals or the public. Therefore, this essay will report these findings in some detail.

Recent studies have confirmed the impact of marijuana on memory. Free recall is invariably impaired. Short-term memory is worsened. Inappropriate memories may intrude themselves into consciousness. A wide variety of cognitive tests have demonstrated that the drug compromises speech, thought, attention, and the integration of sensory information. In large amounts, tetrahydrocannabinol (THC) will frequently induce a dreamlike reverie or a paranoid thinking style. Hemispheric dominance shifts to the right hemisphere under cannabis, but this is owing to left hemispheric decrements, not to an improvement in right hemispheric functioning. Sequencing events in time becomes distorted, and this leads to a breakdown of temporal organization.

The desire and energy to work productively are impaired not only during the intoxicated period, but, for chronic users, during the sober interval also. Although simple repetitive tasks may be performed fairly well under marijuana, more complex work is definitely adversely affected.

One of the more important findings for industrial operations is that serious skills impairment can be measured for more than 10 hours after a single marijuana cigarette. This is long after the "stoned" state has disappeared and the person feels normal. These studies were done, furthermore, with what would now be called low-grade marijuana, namely with 1 or 2 percent THC cigarettes.

Many requirements for effective human interactions, whether with other humans or with machines, deteriorate under marijuana. Tracking ability, complex reaction time, hand steadiness, complicated signal interpretation, and attention tasks are examples of psychomotor activities poorly performed under cannabis. The deficiencies in memory, perception, and cognition make learning difficult, a serious handicap in any endeavor, including all but routine work. Pilots who have to orient themselves in three-dimensional space have a particularly difficult time functioning adequately under the influence of marijuana. Although I have no fear of flying, I would be fearful of being in a plane piloted by someone who has used marijuana within the past day.

Using vehicle operation as an example of a frequently performed skilled occupational activity, and one comparable to the operation of many industrial machines, one can only say that intoxication with marijuana is as impairing as alcohol intoxication.

A study of blood samples from fatally injured drivers in Ontario revealed that 3 percent of the dead drivers had THC in their blood. We know that THC disappears from the blood rapidly, within 20 to 30 minutes if the usual commercial laboratory techniques are employed. This would suggest that marijuana-intoxicated drivers are overrepresented in fatal accidents. Twelve percent of the deceased had THC in their urine. When the accidents were studied to determine who was at fault, the probability of responsibility for the collision was as great for those who had THC metabolites in their urine as for those who had alcohol in their blood. This suggests that marijuana is as potentially dangerous as alcohol in the operation of a motor vehicle. The combination of alcohol and cannabis is more dangerous than either alone, as might be expected.

LEGAL ISSUES

A number of legal issues arise when substance abuse is suspected on the job, or urine testing becomes a matter of company policy for pre-employment physicals.

Testing for Cause

It is well established that an employer can request a urine screen (which tests for the commonly abused substances) when an employee's performance is impaired. If it is positive, and the presence of a drug is confirmed by a second laboratory method, certain actions might be taken. Referral to an employee assistance program or disciplinary action are two options. Possible legal problems include:

1. Violation of contract. Although some unions have cooperated with management on the urine-testing question, others have insisted that unless urine screens were specifically written into the bargaining agreement, they could not be performed. This objection was sustained when a railroad company attempted to do breath alcohol tests on their engineers.

2. Negligence actions. If evidence of improper laboratory performance, chain of custody procedures, or reporting test results can be proven to be faulty, negligence actions are possible.

3. Invasion of employee privacy. While the question of inquiring into employee conduct that affects job performance has not been questioned, the rights of employee behavior off the job are probably protected by constitutional privacy rights. The matter of positive marijuana (actually THC metabolites) urine tests and deficient job performance has special difficulties because the test may remain positive for days (or weeks if a more sensitive test is used) after smoking one marijuana cigarette.

4. Pre-employment screening. It is generally believed that job applicants can be tested for drugs, although certain government employees and related groups may be protected by antidiscrimination laws against the handicapped. Applicants may not be denied employment solely because they are drug abusers in some instances.

Means of Avoiding Legal Problems

1. Employees should have advance notice that illegal drug use is a ground for dismissal.

2. Employers should write employment contracts that permit drug testing when job performance is impaired.

3. The testing laboratory must follow the test manufacturer's instructions precisely, particularly when confirmation of a positive test is recommended.

4. The usual disciplinary channels should be used, including hearings and union representation.

5. Job applicants should be notified of the testing, and they should consent in writing. They should be told that disqualification will occur if the tests are positive. The job's requirement for mental alertness and clarity should be documented.

6. A relationship between the detrimental effect of drug abuse and the job should be provided, for example, in occupations involving public safety, public trust, or the need for precision workmanship.

7. Routine testing of all employees is not likely to be permitted under current statutes unless a clear relationship is demonstrated between drug abuse and the need for unimpaired job performance. As with testing for cause, labor-management contracts should be written to include routine or random testing.

BIBLIOGRAPHY

- Ferraro, D.P. Acute effects of marijuana on human memory and cognition. In: *Marijuana: Research Findings, 1980,* Ed.: R.C. Petersen, U.S. Government Printing Off., Washington, D.C. 20402, 1980.
- Neincek, R.G. Marijuana in the workplace. In: *Drug Abuse in the Modern World: A Perspective for the Eighties.* Eds.: G.G. Nahas and H.C. Frick, Pergamon, New York, 1982, pp. 121–126.
- Vicary, J.R. and Resnik, H. *Preventing Drug Abuse in the Workplace.* DHSS Publication No. (ADM) 82–1220, 1982.

40. The Problem of Acute Affluence: The High-Priced Athlete

Whom the Gods would destroy, they first
endow with sudden wealth.
——*Anonymous*

Although we envy the persons who abruptly strike it rich, a study of their subsequent careers indicates that many of their lives are far from idyllic. This is particularly true of spectacularly successful professional sports figures or entertainers. In addition to the need to manage an immense cash flow, they must cope with a name and face that everyone recognizes and with the accompanying heady adulation. The combination of instant wealth and fame can be overwhelming. It can lead to personal disasters for those not quite wise enough to avoid the many pitfalls of success.

THE DISORDERS OF SUDDEN AFFLUENCE AND THE ATHLETE

The disorders of sudden affluence are manifold, but only the pharmacologic problems that confront the athlete will be discussed here. Most people have fantasized about becoming a star athlete, and they have assumed that this would be the best of all possible worlds. For some athletes it is, but others are unable to deal with the abrupt lifestyle shift from rags to riches. Sports figures are supposed to maintain the macho image of the hard drinking, carousing man's man. Meanwhile a bevy of clever hustlers are on a constant vigil to rip them off.

Certain pressures, not readily apparent to those who envy them, confront the star. There are pressures to party, pressures to continue to excel at their sport, and the stresses of separation from family, boredom, and loneliness. Being in the limelight, gratifying though it is at first, can become a drag. Alternatively, it gives the athlete an inflated image of himself.

SOCIAL IMPLICATIONS

Since outstanding athletes are in the public eye, their comportment and public behavior affect the fan's attitudes. This is especially true for the youngster whose adulation of sports heroes borders on worship. It is true that athletes need not devote their existence to being positive role models. Nevertheless they must be aware of the influence they exert upon adolescents for good or ill. When such heroic figures are seen or reported as drunks or drug addicts, the ramifications extend beyond any harm to the player and the team, extending out to the fans, and especially the youngsters.

We all share some of the blame for a situation in which players must perform beyond their maximum in order to win. The fans must share the responsibility for insisting that winning no matter what the cost is the goal. This attitude can lead to the use of various chemicals presumed to improve performance. The owner, manager, and coaches cannot ignore or trivialize substance abuse and should not permit badly injured players to continue exposing themselves to additional damage.

A well-thought-out policy of prevention, detection, and treatment should be instituted by management. Continuing the destructive use of drugs or relapse after an effort at rehabilitation is a sign of failure, and it cannot be rewarded by retaining the player in the hope that it will go away. It should be understood by the players and their unions that serious infractions like dealing or the inability to remain abstinent despite professional assistance, require automatic dismissal. The players, of course, have the greatest responsibility of all concerned to avoid overdrinking or drug abuse. If they do become involved, they must know that there is one and only one chance—to be rehabilitated. Since physical and mental well-being are their greatest resources, they should be protected from impairment by chemicals.

COCAINE AND THE ATHLETE

It is unusual to read through the sports section of a metropolitan newspaper these days and not find a mention of drug or alcohol misuse. Either some athlete has been found dealing, using, or acting in an unusual manner, or he or she has taken a cure. Urine testing is often debated in the media. Commissioners are repeatedly issuing press releases about cleaning up their league.

Only three years ago when the first essay on drugs in sports was written, little mention was made of cocaine. (See *The Substance Abuse Problems*, pp. 352-357.) Amphetamines were the preferred stimulants of that day, preferred for increasing aggressiveness and alertness and for diminishing the pain of injuries. Although amphetamines have by no means disappeared, cocaine has rapidly come into prominence recently as a "social" stimulant, pregame "lift," and gametime energizer.

It is odd that cocaine snorting is preferred to produce hyperalertness during a game since its duration of action is so brief that it cannot be trusted to last through any sports contest except, perhaps, a mile run. To stay up on cocaine during a football game would require a number of snorts. Even using again at halftime would not cover the entire period of play. If the player tried to extend the effective time of cocaine by snuffling a large amount, it could overstimulate and distort his judgment and performance. What probably happens is that cocaine is snorted on the sidelines from containers that automatically measure out a "line."

Cocaine used in a compulsive manner, even if rarely used on the ballfield, can reduce playing ability. Cocaine binges or consistent, frequent use lead to loss of weight, insomnia, but above all, preoccupation with cocaine and mental disorganization. Concentration on other activities, including one's work, becomes increasingly difficult and eventually impossible.

Highly paid athletes are more vulnerable than the rest of us to compulsive cocaine use in at least one respect. The economic deterrent does not exist for them. If it costs $1,000.00 or so a day to maintain a sizable cocaine habit, not many of us can afford such expenditures and therefore we are not at risk. But the high-priced star can.

ALCOHOL AND THE ATHLETE

Problem drinking is a high risk activity among professional athletes. It is not really to be included in the disorders of affluence because almost everyone can somehow obtain enough beverage alcohol to become an alcoholic.

The tales of enormous drinking bouts before a game by pros, and their ability to perform excellently later, tend to be barroom exaggerations. A superlative player might be able to manage such a feat, but not for long. Even after the alcohol is all eliminated, and only the hangover lingers on, functioning is demonstrably worsened. Many a career has been shortened or terminated by heavy drinking. Fortunately, those in trouble are coming forward for help, and more team organizations have established rehabilitation policies.

After retirement from the game another danger period exists. The spotlight is gone and life may be less interesting. In fact, unless the retirement is planned, it may be empty and boring. A frequent solution to the loss of the glory and the fame is overdrinking.

URINE TESTING

The entire problem of drug/alcohol abuse could be quite easily resolved if we adopted the Olympic or foreign professional soccer league requirement that every contestant must submit urine specimens at the end of a competition.

This has practically eliminated the use of mind-altering drugs by the contestants in these games. We have not adopted urine testing except in isolated instances on the ground that it constitutes an infringement of one's personal freedom. If the drug/alcohol problem were a minor one, it would be unnecessary and undesirable to institute the costly and elaborate laboratory procedure. But at this time, when cocaine and other drugs are fairly widely used, it seems indicated. Otherwise, the practice spreads, and sport contests become a game of competing chemicals, not of humans.

The loss of personal freedom issue has to be considered. It is not the loss of freedom to ingest whatever drug one wants. That freedom does not exist in this country or in any other nation in the world. What it seems to be is a loss of the freedom not to supply a sample of one's urine, a trivial freedom considering the benefits to be derived. It is not a demeaning act if the results are used in the context of improving the health of the individual athlete. Agreements would have to be written to include management's right to request and obtain such material just as they have the right to obtain X rays and blood samples. Other, less well-paid organizations like the armed forces have such regulations. Certain industries have or are considering similar contractual agreements. Higher courts have not ruled on the precise problem.

Urine-testing programs would deter use and identify users so that evaluation of and assistance to the player can be provided. False positives, finding a positive test in someone who is not using drugs, is a rarity when confirmatory tests are automatically performed on all positives. False negatives, not finding the drug on testing after it has been used, is more likely. Although a user may occasionally succeed in passing one urine test, it is not likely that he or she will succeed in passing a second or a third test.

It all depends on what is considered a positive. If the cutoff point of THC metabolites, for example, is placed at 100 nanograms per milliliter of urine, then only moderate or heavy users are likely to be found positive on a gas chromatography confirmatory test. If lower cutoff levels are used, more false positives and fewer false negatives will result.

SUMMARY

The increasing commercialism of the sports industry has produced a new set of demands upon the athletes concerned and upon the managerial group. The exponential increase in salaries of the first rank players is difficult for young men and women to sensibly deal with. Drugs, including alcohol, are readily available solutions to the various pressures and stresses to which the athlete is exposed on and off the playing field. The drug solution inevitably becomes a greater problem than the original problem it was supposed to resolve.

41. Pleasure and Pain

It is surprising that mood alterations, the principal reason why drugs are abused, have not been more carefully studied. The powerful reinforcing properties of pleasurable sensations and the relief of psychological pain initiate and perpetuate the protracted use of mind-altering drugs. If this is so, then a more intensive scrutiny of the numerous elements subsumed under the terms "pleasure" and psychic distress or "pain" could be helpful in dealing with destructive drug use.

MYTHS ABOUT EUPHORIA

At the outset it is necessary to demolish a few erroneous notions that we have unthinkingly adopted. The first of these is that every society has its culturally accepted euphoriant. Although many social systems do, some do not, and even where a majority do indulge in some legal and widely used mood-changer, a minority will remain abstinent. A number of social and religious communities interdict tranquilizing and altering potions. Moslems, Mormons, and Seventh Day Adventists are examples. So it appears that humans do not inevitably require external pacifiers to endure. However, there are those who are swamped by what seem to be ordinary stresses of living and others who sink under the pressures of overwhelming existential catastrophes. But perhaps we should talk not of dysphoric crises but of the simple ability to enjoy. Here, too, some of us can savor this life, and others are unable to know sober delight. Apparently, endogenous receptor sites and their ligands exist that modulate our ability to endure anxiety and dread.

We know that pleasure and displeasure centers are to be found in the posterior hypothalamus. My point is that despite the widespread use of mood-changing chemical configurations, a biologic need for them does not exist in most people.

Another legend asserts that since some tribe or culture used an indigenous plant to alter consciousness without adverse effects, therefore other cultural groups can safely adopt such an item. The reasoning goes: since coca leaves are chewed by the Andean Indians, why not cocaine in Hollywood? Or, if opium is smoked in Southeast Asia, why not in San Francisco? The error in such thinking is bifurcated. First, strict rituals have evolved in established rural societies to protect the user from excessive use. Often such mind-moving agents are used in a religious context on special ceremonial occasions, like the peyote or the psilocybe mushroom rites. When their use is transposed to an entirely different society, without the protecting rituals and taboos, the results can be devastating. Secondly, coca cannot be equated with cocaine, and when the latter is delivered by placement into a vein, the reaction is so different from coca leaf chewing that it virtually becomes a different drug.

Then there is the claim that we should have the freedom to use whatever consciousness-changing chemicals we wish. At first glance this idea seems tenable. Szasz[1] has stated: "I believe that just as we regard freedom of speech and religion as fundamental rights, so should we also regard freedom of self-medication." Arguing this point, not on the visible public health grounds, but rather on civil libertarian grounds, I can only disagree.[2] The loss of freedom from the usage of euphoriants can be considerable. Many of these drugs eventually produce physical dependence, an unhappy state associated with major losses of personal freedom. One is locked into a connection and a supply of the drug. Addiction has been called slavery, but such words are not fashionable anymore. But consider what it means to somehow obtain increasing amounts of some expensive psychochemical daily, every day. Another constriction of personal freedom is the requirement that consistent hedonic drug use demands a major part of one's existence.

It is rather difficult, but not impossible, to support a substantial drug habit from one's own resources. Fair numbers of people are forced to obtain funds illegally or in ways that are distinctly unpleasant. There are cocaine-dependent individuals who have sold everything, stolen from relatives and friends, and who will do anything, really anything, to get one more fix.

THE NATURE OF "HIGH"

The ubiquitous word "high" is used to describe a positive altered mental state produced by drugs. "High" is a collective word with many divergent meanings to users. We should not accept it as descriptive of what takes place. It is necessary to penetrate into the meaning of the word so that an understanding of what the drug experience means to each individual can be acquired.

1. "High" may be used to describe a feeling of well-being, or as Huxley[3] said in his *Doors of Perception*, of "allrightness."

2. The disinhibitory effects of the drug may be perceived as enjoyable. Ego controls over thoughts and behavior are relaxed. Self-monitoring and

self-criticism are reduced so that one's verbal or motor performance seems better than ever.

3. A diminution of drive states is experienced as pleasing, especially if conflicts about the drives had existed previously.

4. Variations in the level of awareness are sought after. These shifts may be in the direction of either a stimulated hyperalertness and increased sensitivity to sensory input, or an obtunded, stuporous state with a distancing from environmental stimuli.

5. Certain drugs induce feelings of mastery and power, sometimes even omnipotence, and these are valued, particularly by people who have doubts about their own competency.

6. Those with high levels of shyness, boredom, loneliness, or tension will find temporary relief in a variety of psychochemicals. As a matter of fact, they will obtain so much more relief than less distraught persons that as a group they are more likely to become overinvolved in excessive drug use. This constitutes an effort at self-treatment, and self-treatment with psychoactive agents is always tricky because supervision is not available to avoid the pitfalls of overdose, dependence, or the distortions of judgment induced by some drugs.

7. Another group who may obtain marked, transient relief and who are therefore vulnerable to become chronic users are aphoric (or anhedonic) individuals. They are unable to feel any emotion strongly and have difficulties in forming warm, meaningful relationships with others. Under the influence of alcohol or some other drug they "feel more like people."

So "high" means several things: euphoric relaxation from the cares of the day, awayness, decreased self-observation, attenuation of drives and reduced guardedness. It can mean surcease from suffering and other dysphoric feelings. It may also procure a short holiday from a painful aphoria in those unable to generate pleasurable feelings from within. Knowing which aspects of "high" are important to our patients will assist us in planning their rehabilitation.

NATURAL VS. CHEMICAL PLEASURES

When people relate pleasurable experiences that occurred either naturally or while under the influence of some drug, many similarities can be identified. But there are differences. The mood swings may be even more extreme in the drugged condition. Elated and ecstatic feelings following the CNS stimulants or the hallucinogens are more reminiscent of mania than of spontaneous happiness.

One striking difference between the two pleasure states is the ephemeral quality of the chemical "high." It is insubstantial and fades quickly. For cocaine the "high" can be counted in minutes. Recall of the "high" during the sober interval does not bring back any of the experienced gladness, and no cocaine user has claimed to learn how to be "high" without cocaine. In contrast, joyful events achieved during an act of creation, interpersonal love, or some other exhilarating activity are often remembered along with some resurgence of the original emotion. In the latter sequence of events the many associational elements surrounding the joyful happening provide a multidimensional quality. It is richer, more meaningful than a chemically induced one. So it is joyful relationships, not contentless joy, that enrich living and sustain us during difficult times.

Chemical enjoyment is not associated with an object—except the chemical itself. The contentless giggles of certain marijuana experiences are examples of objectless enjoyment. On the other hand, ordinary pleasures are intermeshed with a person, a place, or an activity. This gives internally generated pleasures an added dimension that can hardly be approached with drugs.

Drugs do not teach us how to live more gratifying, enjoyable lives. It is for this reason that those who use drugs to manage their serious emotional or personality problems are never helped, except briefly. We do not learn through drugs how to resolve the problems that make us unhappy; in fact, often enough drugs exacerbate life problems.

THE NEUROPHYSIOLOGIC LIMITS TO JOY

A temporary escape from the hassles and tumults of existence can hardly be condemned so long as no harm is done to oneself or others. Occasional fun achieved with chemicals might be acceptable if only we also learn, or do not forget, how to enjoy on our own resources. The trouble is that the chemical "high" becomes an end in itself, and when its use becomes intense, acquiring the strategies needed to deal with life are arrested, and psychological maturation may never occur. This could be the reason why adolescents seem to be more impaired by intoxicants than more mature adults.

There are other problems. Consider De Quincey's[4] paean in praise of his first encounter with opium. "Happiness might now be bought for a penny [things were cheaper in those days] and carried in the waistcoat pocket, portable ecstasies might be corked up in a pint bottle, and peace of mind could be sent down by the mail." Ah, but later, tolerance, dependency, withdrawal, loss of creative ability, family disruption, and something which in that day was called "ruin," emerged.

It is not unusual to escalate the use of a drug that provides euphoria, early to explore its higher reaches, later in the career because of the onset of tolerance. The difficulty is that offering the brain more is not necessarily better. With cocaine and amphetamines, one slips from euphoria into a distressing dysphoria at the upper ranges. Beyond that, paranoid psychoses can come forth. With the CNS depressants, the euphoria gives way to a drunken state often accompanied by negative-feeling tones. Chronic use likewise will flip the emotional response toward dysphoria. After narcotic addiction has set in, the drug is used, often enough, to evade the aversive effects of withdrawal rather than in expectation of the original "high." At this point a paradox exists: the opiate is used to feel normal rather than euphoric.

As repetitively used stimulants leave the brain, the "high" disappears and the mood drops well below the baseline so that the user feels sad, dejected, depressed (the coke blues). This biphasic action on mood is the neurophysiologic price we pay. It can be an important factor in drug-seeking behavior. The user knows that another dose of the stimulant will "cure" the dysphoria. Therefore, it is most unusual for the intravenous cocaine user or the freebaser to stop before the supply has been completely consumed. Then comes the "crash." The cyclic pattern of extreme "highs" that is followed by painful "lows" locks the user into a craving for more drug that can defy the best of intervention efforts.

Incessant electrical stimulation of the nonspecific reward centers in the posterior hypothalamus induces a refractory period during which further stimulation produces no pleasurable response. It appears that continuing chemical stimulation over the dopaminergic pathways to these same centers also results in first a waning and then a nonresponsiveness to what should be pleasurable. This takes place either because the neurotransmitter is eventually depleted or because receptor cell sensitivity is lost. It would be most interesting and clinically relevant to know whether such prolonged chemical stimulation alters the usual threshold setting of the receptors. Would ordinarily pleasurable events become less so? Will the ability to enjoy nonchemical pleasures decrease for an extended period of time? This testable hypothesis should be studied one day, because if the threshold for the reward centers were to remain elevated, then this would be another reason for an increased use of pharmacologic euphoriants.

SUMMARY

It is unlikely that hedonic drug consumption will ever recede to the levels of a half century ago. The use of a number of culture-alien euphoriants has become almost institutionalized, and many of the traditional prohibitions, for example, the use of a needle to inject oneself or the dealing in drugs, have vanished among some middle-class folks. What we can hope for is that some will turn to more sustaining ways to achieve pleasure and more effective ways to manage unpleasure.

REFERENCES

1. Szasz, T.S. The ethics of addiction. Amer. J. Psychiat. 128: 541–546, 1971.
2. Cohen, S., A Commentary on "The ethics of addiction." Amer. J. Psychiat. 128: 547–550, 1971.
3. Huxley, A. *The Doors of Perception*. New York, Harper & Row, 1954.
4. De Quincey, T. *Confessions of an English Opium Eater*. Harper & Row, New York, 1932.

42. Reflections on People and Drugs

Once in a while it is helpful to stand apart from our immediate and urgent problems involving the abuse of substances. A brief period of reflection about the more universal elements conducive to the drugged state might make the clinical anarchy and the informational confusion that confront us a bit more understandable.

The fact that large numbers of humans place nonnutrients into their orifices is a phenomenon shared by few other species. True, a barroom dog can be trained to become a lush, and with modern technology, animals can be converted into insatiable cocaine consumers. Even in nature, tales exist of wild horses deliberately eating locoweed, or of elephants seeking out the fallen, fermented fruit of overripe prunus species, but these are rarities.

The use of medicines seems to be almost exclusively a human characteristic. The discovery of medications for pain or dread is life sustaining. The consumption of botanicals or their derivatives for intoxication is essentially a humanoid trait and, indeed, an ancient one. What can be said of the deliberate intoxication of the mind, a condition resulting in a temporarily diminished survival capability? Is it true, as some claim, that man's predicament is so deplorable that sustained sober awareness is not possible?

SOME NOTIONS ABOUT THE HUMAN CONDITION

1. All vertebrates, and many nonvertebrates, are able to sense pain and fear. Animals like dolphins and some primates are able to conceptualize the future and have some level of self-awareness. Among these primates are the hairless and tailless humans who seem to be unfinished organisms in that they have real difficulties in adapting to unease, stress, boredom, unhappiness, ambiguity, etc. Anxiety, that is, fear without a specific cause, and depression are maladaptive responses that are common mortal experiences.

2. Human consciousness permits self-awareness, self-scrutiny, and future

239

orientation. People are aware of their mortality and the inevitability of extinction. Consciousness is an extraordinary gift but an unsettling one.

3. Like all animals, including one-celled animals and some plants, people try to move away from noxious stimuli and toward pleasant ones. Exceptions to this universal tropism exist. For example, people will often forgo pleasure now if displeasure later is a perceived consequence. And a few, for idiosyncratic motives, will prefer punishments to rewards.

THE DRUG/HUMAN INTERACTION

With the above concepts in mind, the drug/human interaction can be examined with particular reference to intoxicant/euphoriant substances. Many cultures, past and present, have used a wide variety of intoxicants, almost invariably of plant origin. Not all societies have employed drugs for this purpose; in fact, a substantial minority, perhaps even a majority of the world's population, does not seek chemical mind alteration. Availability is one reason for abstinence, but religious, moral, and political interdictions persuade large numbers to forgo such experiences. When large populations of abstainers are studied, their ability to deal with catastrophes and to enjoy life's pleasures is no less than that of groups who use mind-changing drugs. The point that every culture has and requires an intoxicant seems to be a rationalization of those who use them.

On the other hand, chemical inducers of euphoria have been so widely sought after that some great need for them must exist. It may be, as suggested, that we are an incompletely developed, maladapted species. An alternative proposition must be considered: that we are bent on altering our environment so rapidly and drastically that adaptation becomes hardly possible. History lends some support to both hypotheses.

WHAT'S NEW AND DIFFERENT?

A quarter century ago we moved from a low-level usage of marijuana, opiates, and other assorted oddities to a widespread preoccupation with LSD among young adults. The drug scene has continued and changed, never completely dropping the original items, but adding new drugs or reviving half-forgotten ones. To list some of the more prominent: speed, heroin, marijuana, newer solvents like the volatile nitrites, phencyclidine, methaqualone, tranquilizers, and during the past five years, cocaine.

As we try to understand the psychochemical gyrations of these past two decades, it is evident that what started out as a search for inner meaning and "mind expansion" has long since deteriorated into a search either for "high" or mind reduction. This decaying course is common in all revolutions, chemical and nonchemical, and lest we forget, in the 1960s the psychedelic revolution was loudly proclaimed. What ever happened to the psychedelic revolution?

But novel and unique aspects of our current drug picture should be listed.

1. For the first time in history, very young people are the most heavily involved group. For both psychologic and physiologic reasons, youth may be the group least able to use chemicals for the mind wisely or well.

2. The drugs are more potent, and the delivery systems are more efficient. The trend toward increasing potency will continue. Narcotics a hundred times more powerful than heroin are known. Intravenous cocaine is nothing new, but the numbers of "mainliners" have increased. Inhaling the vapors of cocaine base competes with the intravenous route for speed of delivery to the brain. The marijuana is stronger, but to counter the trend, light beers and lower-proof whiskeys have appeared in the marketplace.

3. Never before in history have we witnessed concurrent or sequential multiple drug use in which bemusing combinations of agents are introduced into the body.

These are all unfavorable indicators, unfavorable for the individual and for the public. In attempting to understand how these new developments in the abuse of drugs relate back to fundamental human conditions, we can hypothesize the following.

1. Too many people are utilizing poor adaptive responses to life stress and are attempting to resolve problems and dysphoria with a drug or drugs. Learning to deal with adversity is more sustaining and more successful.

2. Conceptualizing the future and attention to one's body and mind are diminished. If our evolution lies in the direction of greater consciousness and awareness, then drug intoxication and euphoria run counter to our destiny.

3. Drug hedonism is an excellent example of the hedonic paradox. Our central nervous system is wired for pleasure, and our training reinforces the movement toward the pleasurable. Rewards for eating, drinking, and sex are built in for survival as an individual and a species. Other rewarding activities: creating, learning, problem solving, and relating to others have a second order survival value and are considered to be desirable human activities. They also tickle the reward centers of the brain. Pleasure for pleasure's sake—entertainment, for example—is accepted and widely indulged in. Many drugs provide initial pleasure, and when used moderately may continue to provide

pleasurable feelings. This does not mean that even a single exposure to a drug may not produce negative consequences: overdose, accidents, mental disturbances, and so forth. What is paradoxical is that an important minority of users of any psychoactive drug becomes overinvolved in that drug. This is either because tolerance and withdrawal symptoms drive the person back to the drug, or because the pleasurable state induces compulsive use. At these points, the rewards diminish and the punitive aspects of the drug dominate. What began as a pleasurable practice has, because of neurophysiologic events in the brain, become the opposite.

We can do no more than guess who will be trapped into dysphoric drug experiences. With unlimited access to a drug like cocaine, perhaps everyone is vulnerable. Human evolution has advanced to the stage where certain pleasures can be delayed or denied because longer term displeasure can exceed whatever immediate pleasure is experienced. Without this ability the social fabric frays.

43. The Now People: Sketches of Lethal Drug Use

A trait, almost exclusively human, is to look ahead, to include estimates of the future in our present plans and acts. That future may be only as distant as tomorrow for some, while others may think in terms of 20-year plans and beyond.

A related human characteristic, widely shared by other species, is the desire to survive, the so-called survival instinct. Future orientation and survival are so deeply ingrained in our conceptual style that we are hardly aware of them. When we come upon instances of overt self-destructive behavior, they are often difficult to understand and impossible to explain.

On the other hand it's not possible to lead a completely safe life. A wide variety of not-so-safe activities is indulged in by all. Every day we take a series of low-grade risks, without which life would be intolerably boring or almost impossible. We cross streets, ride in cars, fly in airplanes, climb ladders, and engage in contact sports. The totally risk-free life is difficult to visualize, and it would not be a very attractive sort of existence. It might be assumed that spending one's life in bed may constitute the optimum in playing it safe but cardiac physiologists tell us that the completely sedentary life also has its dangers.

Then there is a group of high-risk takers who willingly expose themselves to danger for the exhilaration of other rewards of the risk taking. There are the sky divers, the motorcycle and car racers, members of bomb disposal units, and others who knowingly engage in similar hazardous avocations or vocations for money or fun.

So we all live in ways that will predictably shorten our life span. Many of our habits of eating, drinking, smoking, and other ventures are not likely to procure the longest possible survival. Lack of exercise, obesity, overdrinking, or heavy smoking are fairly likely to shorten one's existence, but fair numbers of us seem willing to accept that contingency. This disregard for longevity is probably a result of the delay in the perceived result. Disregarding the possibility of a shortened existence is not hard if the ultimate consequences are years away. Couched in terms of learning theory, consequences that are immediate and pleasurable or pain relieving are much more reinforcing of behavior than consequences that are distant and aversive.

THE NOW PEOPLE

Over and above the "normal" disregard for maximal survival, certain people seem to have little or no concept of a personal future. They become involved in life-threatening behaviors because they cannot conceive of their own cessation. In general, adolescents tend to be now oriented and often behave as though they were immortal. In fact, the end of psychological adolescence may coincide with the first shocking awareness of one's own mortality. A few adults never seem to have acquired this insight and continue to act as though they were imperishable. Their lifestyle reflects a singular lack of concern about their continuance.

Then there are those who exist without a viable future. In reality or in their fantasy—it doesn't matter which—they are without hope. Their emotional condition ranges from dysphoria to aphoria. Such noxious feeling tones demand relief, no matter that the relief is achieved at a perilous price.

Finally, the now people include those who have been tricked into futurelessness. Some chemical, taken over time, reduces or obliterates the ability to know the consequences of its continued consumption. Alternatively, one may become locked into a drug's repetitive use because of the withdrawal sickness that is so easily relieved by the substance that caused the sickness. It is fascinating to observe certain otherwise thoughtful people advocate the right to unlimited access to all drugs as a basic freedom when, in fact, dependence on certain drugs drastically impairs or abolishes one's freedom of choice.

It is not surprising that a number of the now people eventually seek out certain mind-altering drugs that will make them feel better than they do. It is also not surprising that such drugs will be excessively used, either because the degree of relief provided is great, or because the usual internal constraints and cultural taboos hardly exist for these people.

The now people do not see any reason why they should not continue to use, and why they should not use as much as they need to provide hyperphoria. They are not the experimenters or the recreational users of drugs. They make a career of their substance abuse. They are the rumheads, the potheads, the pillheads, and the hopheads. And their inordinate drug consumption serves to reinforce their futurelessness.

LETHAL PATTERNS OF DRUG ABUSE

Most drug abuse has no lethal intent. Nonmedical drug users as a group are quite concerned about their viability and survivability.

One example of their concern for themselves was the loud outcry about Mexican marijuana being contaminated by the herbicide paraquat. In fact, there has not yet been a substantiated instance of paraquat toxicity due to marijuana use. That whole uproar was a tempest in a waterpipe, more political than pathological.

But there are certain highly hazardous drug-using practices. Some of them are well known; some are insufficiently documented because the research has not been done, but the street reports are ominous. It is a remarkable commentary on our alleged "instinct for survival" that these precarious patterns of drug abuse are not too uncommon. A number of them will be mentioned to illustrate the self-destructive inclinations of those who have, for one reason or another, little concern about their future.

THE END-STAGE, ACTIVELY DRINKING ALCOHOLIC

The person in, or verging on, liver failure who continues to drink is unquestionably hastening his or her demise. By this time he or she must have been told repeatedly of the grim consequences of the continued ingestion of alcoholic beverages. People who have had portocaval shunts for bleeding varices or ascites have been known to continue to imbibe.

I can think of at least one person with a severe alcoholic peripheral neuritis that rendered him incapable of walking, who managed to push his wheelchair to the nearest liquor store for a daily jug of wine. Then there was the relatively young man with recurrent bouts of acute alcoholic pancreatitis associated with excruciating abdominal pain who would resume drinking shortly after discharge from the hospital. One might have thought that the immediate and obvious threat of dying or of inordinate suffering would be a deterrent. But it was not.

THE PHENCYCLIDINE FREAK

PCP is a rather mediocre euphoriant, but it is widely available, and the price is right. As a result, the young in mind who are despairing, distraught, distressed, desolate, or depressed have come to use the drug often and in increasing amounts. Too often one of a variety of lethal sequallae emerges. Overdose, with death from recurrent seizures or respiratory failure, is one possibility. Accidental drowning from loss of orientation, sometimes in small amounts of water, is another. A third is violence to oneself or to others, or deadly force used upon the "dusted" person whose aggressiveness induces counterviolence. A suicidal depression can emerge after partial recovery from a major phencyclidine reaction.

One of the strangest of angel dust-related phenomena is the repeated use of the drug after experiencing a devastating, schizophrenic-like psychosis. It is not a rarity to find that after recovery from one or more psychotic episodes of many weeks' duration, the person decides to continue to use the drug despite the previous devastating experience with it.

THE HOT SHOT

When a heroin user overdoses, it is not unusual for junkies who become aware of the event to try to seek out the pusher who sold the material. They assume that the quality of the heroin must be better than the usual street junk, and they want some. The possibility that they might also OD doesn't seem to deter them.

INHALING THE COMMERCIAL SOLVENTS

The abuse of a drug that has been tested for safety and has been used in medicine is one thing. To sniff organic solvents that have never been meant to be used by man or beast reflects a profound disinterest in survival. Not only the solvent, but also the impurities and the active ingredients may be toxic. Such exotic items as insecticide spray, liquid shoeshine polish, transmission fluid, and metallic paint aerosols are in favor in certain parts of the country. Even relatively nontoxic solvents can cause death by asphyxiation when sniffed in an enclosed space or by "sudden sniffing death" when inhalation is combined with physical exertion. Now people are never deterred from using dangerous drugs by giving them information about the possible consequences.

SPEED ROULETTE

As the intravenous speed scene was drawing to a close, about 1970, an occasional tale was heard of two or more speedfreaks competitively injecting large amounts of methamphetamine. They would each mainline teaspoons of methamphetamine every hour or so. The winner was the one who could walk away. Whatever happened to the speedfreaks?

THE TOILET WATER FIX

One scene that remains etched in my memory occurred a dozen years ago at Piccadilly Circus, a favorite gathering place for London's heroin addicts. I was in the underground men's room when, through a partly opened door, I saw a young man filling a syringe with water from the toilet bowl. He had apparently obtained sterile syringes and sterile heroin from the nearby pharmacy, yet he preferred the water closet to the cleaner water from the nearby wash basins. I immediately realized why British addicts get hepatitis and other infections as frequently as their American counterparts who do not have access to sterile materials. This young man seemed to have a singular disregard for his well-being.

SMOKE GETS IN MY ARTERIES

Another much more distant memory that will not go away is of a patient who had just been admitted to the surgical service where I was an intern. He had an admitting diagnosis of Buerger's disease (an obliterative disease of the small and medium blood vessels related to heavy smoking) and had amputations, at various levels, of all four extremities. When I asked what brought him into the hospital, he replied with a particular intensity. "I'd like the surgeon to fix a skin flap on my right arm stump so that it will hold a cigarette."

THE "GARBAGEHEAD"

A final reminiscence: during the 1960s when the flower children began moving from the Haight-Ashbury to agrarian communes, I visited one in Northern California to try to understand the new phenomenon. This was a drug-using group who wanted to return to nature while living better through synthetic chemistry. One of the membership was referred to by the others as a "garbagehead."

He would consume any pill or liquid that came his way, known and unknown. He seemed to want only to get away from his ordinary consciousness; it didn't matter how or in which direction.

SUMMARY

Although an immediate survival drive does exist—except in the instance of suicide—a survival instinct that preserves the individual over the long term is not always clearly observable. Those who will shorten or interrupt their lives often are involved in the substance abuse scene, usually as high-dose, compulsive users. Not too much can be done to counteract the overriding need to use drugs perniciously. At the very least, they should be clearly informed of their limited outlook for survival so that ignorance is not a factor in their self-destruction.

The question, of course, is "Why?" Is their drug overuse an unextinguishable behavioral pattern that cannot be broken? Is it a countervailing death instinct? Is it depression or denial? Or is it, indeed, an inability or a refusal to behave as though a personal future existed? The answer remains obscure, but the same in-depth psychodynamic studies should be done with these people as have been performed on suicidal individuals.

44. Drugs for Pleasure: Ethical Issues

Ordinarily, medicines are prescribed to restore people to a state of health, or to prevent certain illnesses from occurring. Physicians also will try to relieve noxious symptoms with drugs, drugs that will obviously not heal or cure.

The abatement of pain, for example, has been considered a desirable goal since the beginnings of medicine. Thus, preventing or treating a disorder or a symptom are the major reasons why drugs are used in medicine.

When we try to understand why drugs are used under nonmedical conditions, the situation is somewhat different. Ask a group of persons why they swallow, inhale, or inject their psychochemical of choice, and the most frequent response is some direct or indirect variant of "to feel better." This reply has two implied meanings. One is that they seek relief from some unpleasant mood, a reduction of their anomie or dysphoria. The distressing mood may be loneliness, boredom, or shyness, but frequently it is a symptom for which doctors often prescribe medicine: tension, depression, or some thought disorder.

A fair number of chronic drug abusers, then, are actually treating themselves for an uncomfortable or disabling psychological condition. Often enough this effort at self-treatment either fails or is replaced by an even more unfortunate situation. Self-treatment with psychoactive medications is always tricky even when the afflicted person is a physician. Supervision is necessary in order to avoid the pitfalls of overdose, dependence, and the distortions of judgment induced by the drug.

The second aspect of "feeling better" is to feel better than they do although they are not in overt physical or mental distress. What they seem to seek is a high—euphoria. The search for euphoria is hardly a new exploration. Through the ages people have been willing to hunt for and try a wide variety of botanicals to achieve a brief interlude of gladness, joy, elation, or simply a respite from the cares of the day. It is said, only partially incorrectly, that each culture has found its own euphoriant. Embedded in the institutionalization of the socially approved euphoriant is, invariably, a set of permissible and pre-scribed rules of usage, and of acceptable and impermissible behaviors in con-nection with its consumption.

One approved euphoriant is, of course, beverage alcohol. Two additional substances need mention: caffeine-containing drinks, and nicotine for those who believe that tobacco is a mind-altering substance. Many other procurers of euphoria have been employed in various societies: opium, cannabis, khat, kava, betel nuts, coca leaves, and dozens of other plants. It must also be noted that the drugs we call hallucinogens, especially when used in lesser dosages, can induce euphoric states. Peyote, caapi, certain South American snuffs, the iboga bean, a few species of morning glory seeds, and the psilocybe mush-room are only a few examples of this class.

THE ETHICS OF CHEMICAL EUPHORIA

A number of questions arise in connection with the use of chemicals to achieve pleasurable states of mind. These questions are particularly relevant at this time when increasing numbers of individuals are utilizing legal and less than legal euphoriants. Furthermore, a quantitative change has occurred in the potency of these materials. The extraction of pure alkaloids and the ability to design synthetic compounds with far greater intensity of psychoactive effects have shifted their effect/side effect ratios. Cocaine is a hundred times stronger than coca leaves, and delivering it into a vein makes it a vastly different drug. Narcotics have been synthesized that are dozens of times more potent than even heroin. We already have amphetamines, barbiturates, and a long list of other compounds that are constructed to activate, depress, or otherwise alter consciousness. These powerful agents are being used without the usual rituals and taboos that ordinarily would protect the members of a tribe from the ad-verse consequences of euphoriant ingestion.

THE PRICE OF PLEASURE

Many religions teach that enjoyment should be earned; it is a reward for virtue, arduous labor, or faith. Freud has written that the ability to delay grati-fication when reality intervenes is an indication of one's maturity. Although joy is only occasionally considered sinful these days, residuals of the notion that we should pay a price for our pleasure remain. Now that, with certain pharmacologic agents or with electrical stimulation of the brain, maximal ac-tivation of the reward (pleasure) centers is possible, the issue becomes more pertinent than ever. Is a state of gratuitous ecstasy equivalent to an ecstatic state achieved spontaneously? Is chemically induced joy to be equated with a similar emotional state that follows an act of creation, interpersonal love, or some other joy-induced activity? What's wrong with instant happiness in pill form?

THE NEUROPHYSIOLOGY OF PLEASURE

There are neurophysiological and personal levels of response to these questions. The nature of neuronal functioning indicates that repetitive and intensive stimulation of the nonspecific reward centers in the posterior hypothalamus by chemical means, eventually results in a diminution of the feeling of elation. More or stronger stimuli are needed to augment the waning emotional response. The neurons involved eventually become refractory to all stimuli. Attempts to prolong these maximal states incessantly will fail; in fact, toxic and dysphoric effects begin to appear. After repetitious chemical highs, it has been noted that the ordinarily pleasurable activities hardly register. The biphasic quality of central nervous system function asserts itself. For each amphetamine run, there follows a postamphetamine depression.

EUPHORIA AND YOU

The personal costs of pleasure procured by chemicals may be considerable. Many of these drugs used eventually produce physical dependence, an unhappy state associated with considerable loss of personal freedom. The user is then condemned to the need to somehow acquire and consume increasing amounts of the drug daily, every day, not only to get high, but also to avoid the distinctly unpleasurable aspects of the withdrawal manifestations. After a while the drug no longer evokes euphoria because of the buildup of tolerance; instead, the chemical must continue to be used to avoid the abstinence syndrome. In other words, it becomes a desperate effort to avoid unpleasure rather than a search for euphoria.

Another constriction upon personal freedom is the requirement that consistent hedonic drug usage demands of one's life style. It is rather difficult—but not impossible—to support a substantial drug habit from one's own resources. Fair numbers of drug-dependent people are forced to obtain funds illicitly or in ways that are distinctly unpleasant. Making all euphoriants legal or even free as some people have suggested will hardly solve the problems of escalating tolerance, of resale of supplies to naive, unaddicted persons, and of the diseases of unsterility when the drugs are injected. If all people were wise, the freedom to use whatever drugs they wished would be a tenable position. Unfortunately that situation does not quite hold at present.

THE INFREQUENT SEEKER AFTER HIGH

What can be said of the occasional, or so-called recreational user who manages to avoid the tolerance trap and does not slip into a lifelong career of searching for chemical euphoria? Such individuals are quite numerous: we do not know their numbers because they are rarely counted in medical or law enforcement registries. The hazards they encounter are far fewer and milder: hangovers, bum trips, poststimulant lows, car accidents, etc.

What is impressive is how unsubstantial the chemically procured highs are. Their staying power is minimal. For cocaine it can be counted in minutes. Recollection of the high state during the sober interval is not associated with a return of the glow. By contrast, joyful events achieved in the course of life experiences are often retrieved with some quality of the original emotion. In the latter sequence of events, the many associational elements of the joyful happening give a multidimensional quality to the memory. It is richer, fuller, more meaningful than the chemically induced one. In fact, one might suggest that the trouble with chemical euphoria is that nothing is learned. It does not teach us how to live more gratifying, enjoyable lives. It is for this reason that those who use such drugs to manage deep emotional or personality problems are hardly ever helped, except momentarily. They do not learn how to deal with the problems that make them feel unhappy. But if the private, infrequent recourse to some instant happiness potion does no harm to the individual or to society, the moral question must be answered according to the specific circumstances.

Nothing is wrong with using a crutch when it is needed as long as it is discarded when it is not. A transient escape from the hassles and tumults of existence can hardly be condemned if, meanwhile, we would learn how to surmount them. Fun, however achieved, is all right so long as it does no harm to oneself or others, and we eventually figure out how to enjoy on our own resources. The trouble is that the chemical high becomes an end in itself, and personal growth may suffer.

DO HUMANS NEED EUPHORIANTS?

The fact that most societies have their approved euphoriants and ataractics makes one wonder whether such agents are necessary in order to endure life as it is. Perhaps, humans have not developed to a level where they can contend with the harsh scrape of reality. Certainly, there are some who are swamped by overwhelming events and others who seem to sink under what seem to be the ordinary stresses of living. But for most, the euphoria producers are not necessary for survival; indeed, they may impair the ability to learn how to survive.

Many social and religious communities do not indulge in mood enhancers. Most Moslems, Mormons, Seventh-Day Adventists and even substantial minorities within societies that use such artifices, have overcome the travails of existence sober at least as well as the users of drugs. Insofar as health and longevity are concerned the Mormons and Adventists have better records than the rest of the population. We do not have good measures of happiness to evaluate what sort of life is more productive of positive emotions.

PERSONAL FREEDOM VS. SOCIAL RESPONSIBILITIES

The perennial ethical dilemma of the reciprocal tensions between our individual freedom and our social responsibility impinges on the use of drugs for mood enhancement. The extreme state of the complete liberty to do as one pleases culminates in anarchy, and complete subservience of the person's well-being to the state becomes totalitarianism. Neither position has much to recommend it.

Certain questions persist. Should individuals have the right to do what they wish to themselves, in this instance the right to use any drug they wish? Does the state have the right to regulate which drugs are to be used and under what specified conditions? In a complex social system like ours, it would appear that the state must take over some of the decision-making process and do so as sagaciously as possible.

The private use of illegal drugs has been called a victimless crime, implying that if only the individual is harmed there is no victim. This libertarian attitude seems short-sighted. Everyone pays for the damage the alcoholic does to himself or herself, to property, and to the life and limbs of others. In particular, the family, close friends, and those in the vicinity of drug dependent people are seriously hurt in a variety of ways. So the assertion that intemperate drug abuse is a victimless crime is specious.

OUR ACCEPTABLE EUPHORIANTS

It is unfortunate that the culturally acceptable euphoriant of the Western world has turned out to be a poor choice from a public health viewpoint. Our society has strongly integrated alcohol into its fabric, and there are few remaining social events where such beverages are not available. Per capita consumption of alcohol increases yearly, and a direct correlation exists between per capita use and the number of problem drinkers.

Alcohol was brought into the culture long before it was possible to study its risks and benefits. Once a substance is incorporated into a civilization, it is extremely difficult or impossible to remove it. The fact that we have an euphoriant-intoxicant with a certain potential for harm is, of course, no reason for introducing new ones.

DISCUSSION

Attempting to analyze our drug situation on ethical rather than on legal grounds provides some interesting perspectives. It is unnecessary to be a "pharmacological Calvinist," a doctorinaire moralist, or a survivor of the Victorian era to find the present-day interminable quest by some for better living through psychochemistry a dubious illusion. The wiring of the brain eventually thwarts attempts to gain perpetual bliss or habitual highs. Nor does the human organism seem to sustain the bedrugged euphoric state without penalties that can exceed the pleasures.

BIBLIOGRAPHY

- Cohen, S. A commentary on "The Ethics of Addiction." Am. J. Psychiat. 128:547–550, 1971.
- Cohen, S. Drug use for pleasure and transcendent experience. In: *Encyclopedia of Bioethics,* Vol. I. Ed.: W.T. Reich, Free Press, New York, 1978, pp. 334–338.
- Neville, R. Drug use, abuse and dependence. In: *Encyclopedia of Bioethics.* Vol. I, Ed.: W.T. Reich, Free Press, New York, 1978, pp. 326--333.
- Veach, R.M. Drugs and competing drug ethics. Hastings Center Report 2(1) 68–80, 1974.

45. Parent Power

For more than a quarter century parenting has become a lost art. Children have often been allowed to grow up on their own, without limit setting and deprived of supervision.

How has this major shift in child rearing come about? In part, it was the lack of child contact and communication with the parents, both of whom may have been employed. Incessant television watching by young people; overpermissiveness; children who treated the home as a pit stop, refueling, and then taking off; parents who were poor role models or had no time—these were some of the reasons for the child-rearing breakdowns. Other reasons existed outside the home: the increased mobility of teenagers, the insensate media, the intensity of peer pressure, and the dissolution of the school as a place where ethical and educational matters were taught.

This lack of control over the young naturally led to its exploitation by them. The astonishing growth of excessive juvenile drug and alcohol use was one important consequence. The current substance abuse crisis is the first in which adolescents and teenagers have been in the vanguard of the mind-altering drug epidemic.

Efforts to deal with this unhappy phenomenon from above downward failed for the most part. Since 1976, a grassroots movement of concerned parents has made a significant contribution in dealing with the problem.

It was an idea whose time had come. A lot of frightened parents around the country were seeing their offspring undergo a blunting of personality, burn out, overdose, kill themselves or others while driving intoxicated on some drug. One parent in Atlanta appears to have ignited the social revolution that resulted in restoring parental guidance and authority in matters that required mature decisions and a consideration of future consequences. Now as many as 5,000 chapters of concerned parents are attempting to cope by preventing their nonusing children from becoming involved and eliminating drug usage when their offspring have become involved. The movement has spread across the land into every social and economic class and is being transplanted to foreign countries.

The major trends that have emerged from observation of the parents' groups are assumption of the parental role and organization of the community.

ASSUMPTION OF THE PARENTAL ROLE

The notion that parents have a responsibility to help their children prepare for the problems of growth in this complex existence is a fundamental premise. With particular reference to alcohol/drug problems it means that, until the age of maturity, and while living under the parental roof, decisions about the use of illegal drugs, intoxication, and related matters are resolved by learning about the agents involved and learning how to solve problems and to arrive at reasonable decisions within the context of the entire family.

This means education about drugs, time spent listening to the children, and developing meaningful, familial activities. The process is not easy for parents or children. For the former it means considerably more time spent within the family; for the latter it means surrendering the "freedom" to indulge, and the requirement to make personal decisions rather than going along with one's peers. Both generations need more self-discipline in their living: the adults must be positive role models in their drinking behavior, the children need to realize that they are neither omnipotent nor indestructible. These changes must be carried out in an evenhanded, wise manner.

The group supports members who are having a particularly difficult time achieving abstinent and reasonable behavior in their children. The concept of tough love is espoused: love and limits.

ORGANIZATION OF THE COMMUNITY

Just as important as organization of the family unit is organization of the parents of the children's friendship group, the schools they attend, and other community groups that are involved in the movement toward reestablishing familial homeostasis. Certain schools have successfully enforced the simple rule: No Drugs. Arrangements with the police are made so that any illegal act is turned over to them. Marked improvement in other irregular activities like truancy, tardiness, and disorderliness are seen as appropriate; uniformly enforced limits are set. Ideally, all relevant community resources are linked with the parent group.

It is impossible for a single family to set up a new, restricting code of conduct for their children if all their friends are still unrestrained and uncontrolled. The children may try to manipulate along the "but all the other kids are doing it" line. Or if they do want to clean up, they will find that remaining a part of their group is difficult or impossible. Therefore most of the parents in the neighborhood should be organized and present a unified set of guidelines of appropriate behavior.

It does not matter whether the parent group focuses on positive parenting approaches in all life areas or concentrates on substance-abusing behavior.

They must eventually deal both with the drug problem and the other problems of surviving.

The national coordinating group, the National Federation of Parents for Drug-Free Youth (NFP), serves to tie the individual community chapters together. It takes positions on legislation and lobbies for their position. One of their notable successes has been the antiparaphernalia bills that have been passed by most state and local jurisdictions and have withstood judicial review.

Parents Resources Institute for Drug Education (PRIDE) at Georgia State University has been an important educational resource, providing instructional materials and holding annual conferences that supply current information on drugs, the parent movement, and family organization.

Much of the emphasis has been on marijuana usage, because marijuana is the illegal drug with which adolescents are most frequently involved. Marijuana (perhaps all psychoactive drugs) are difficult for juveniles to deal with. The adaptive mechanisms for managing intoxication and for avoiding the damaging behavioral consequences of intoxication are not as well developed as in most adults. Some preliminary evidence indicates that the metabolic pathways for degrading drugs and alcohol are not fully functional.

The parent organizations' position on alcohol is that illegal drinking by minors should be prohibited. It is up to the parents if they wish to teach their teenager to drink socially at home.Other consciousness-changing drugs consumed by youth are strongly interdicted, including the look-alikes.

One fallout of the parents movement has been the formation of a number of teenage peer groups that support the same goals. Individuals from these groups can be very effective in changing attitudes toward intoxicants in others of their age. They are not simply against drug use but are for more healthful and enjoyable activities. Many are recovered drug-dependent young people.

DISCUSSION

The rapid growth of the parents' groups indicates that a great need for something like them pre-existed their appearance. A vast submerged source of frustration, anger, and confusion was tapped.

Can such a movement survive? If they succeed in reducing adolescent drug abuse down to a pre-Viet Nam level, they will lose the need for their existence. By that time they will probably have made the transition to much broader goals of enhancing family life styles in America and revivifying the parental role of benign, authoritarian protector and teacher of the young. It is much more likely that success in the "war" against drugs will be partial and that successive generations will be at risk. The need for some sort of network of concerned parents will persist.

The simple wear and tear of going to meetings, volunteer work, and so forth could produce a gradual decline in interest and activity. It is unknown whether there is a birth, maturation, and death cycle to such organizations.

For the underlying principles, a real demand will remain for a long time. A part of the problem has been the strange notion that children should be reared by permissively allowing them to do their thing. Somehow, instinctively, youngsters would know the correct way to grow up. Punishment would serve to inhibit their creative instincts, and only reward was to be used to shape their behavior. This enormous error was foisted on young couples, and the results were chaotic. Without guides, the child naturally attempted to test what the social limits were by seeing how far he or she could go. Neither humans nor other animal species have ever successfully become adults without learning the social and cultural structures and strictures early in life from their elders. In fact, children are harmed by not being taught what is permissible and what is not. They get into trouble trying to find out what is culturally unacceptable. Eventually, they find out from the law enforcement people what is not tolerated.

All sorts of criticisms have been leveled at the parents' organizations. They are too narrow in their approach: dealing with marijuana, and more recently with alcohol and other intoxicants. They are too white, middle class. They read the scientific literature too selectively. They are too authoritarian in their approach. All of these objections do not override the simple fact that they work. They saw their children going to pot, and they wouldn't stand for it. The question of whether or not the amotivational syndrome exists has been answered by their experience. Researchers will go on for decades and come up with a more elegant answer. The present realities could not wait.

What can we derive from parents in action? In addition to the obvious fact that juvenile drug involvement had gone too far, and the responsible people have done something about it, other points have been made. We have learned, or relearned, that one person or a small group of people can make a difference—providing the need exists and the people involved are able to work together and have the ability to organize and persuade. We have learned that attitudes and behaviors can be readily changed, especially in the young, but also in adults.

Despite the success of the family movement, a majority of children and their parents still remain in distress because of drug and alcohol misuse. They are the unorganized families who cannot deal with their problems in the area of substance abuse. How are they to be helped?

SOME ADDRESSES FOR ADDITIONAL INFORMATION

Joyce Nalepka
National Federation of Parents for Drug-Free Youth
1820 Franswell Ave.
Silver Springs, MD 20902

Sue Rusche
Families in Action
3845 N. Druid Hill Road, Suite 300
Decatur, GA 30033

Thomas J. Gleaton, Ed.D.
PRIDE
100 Edgewood Ave, N.E., Suite 1216
Atlanta, GA 30303

VI
AN ASSORTMENT OF ISSUES

46. Drug Abuse: The Coming Years

If the 1960s can be thought of as the upbeat decade of the hyperalerting psychedelics and amphetamines, and the 1970s considered the downbeat period of heroin and the sleepers, what can be said of the 1980s and beyond? If nothing else, it is predictable that drug fashions will change and change again.

At the moment the following situation seems to prevail. Our basic intoxicant, alcohol, maintains its dominance. The trend, though, is toward a lower alcoholic content per dosage unit. Lower proof whiskeys, light beers, and wines are occupying larger proportions of the market.

Most of the other drugs have leveled off or declined in sales volume— drugs like heroin, barbiturates, PCP, LSD, the volatile solvents, and the tranquilizers. Marijuana use also may be on the wane, perhaps because pubescents have appropriated it from their elders, a fatal blow to any drug fad. Alternatively, it may be that the bad news about pot is getting around and having an impact. Marijuana, unlike alcohol, gets stronger. While the ethanol content decreases, the THC percentage increases.

THE COCAINE ERA

But there are exceptions to the standoff in drug usage. If the 1980s will earn a name for itself, it might be: the era of cocaine. Although expensive and adulterated, its impressive ability to tickle the brain's reward centers, plus the rapid delivery systems that have been devised, make it the most compelling drug of all. While fair numbers of snorters can take it or leave it, some are unable to put it down until they or the cocaine are exhausted. As to the freebasing and intravenous crowd, the only real protection they have from their cocaine hunger is insolvency, or the refusal of friends and family to continue to lend or be robbed.

Cocaine drives the user back to cocaine for four reasons, none of which have to do with physical dependence. The first compelling quality is, of course, the euphoria, the feelings of elation, power, and brilliance. The second emerges after a cocaine "run," when the white powder is gone and the sadness, apathy, and dysphoria set in. The cocainist knows (and it is true) that one more "fix" will lift him or her out of the lethargy, at least for a few minutes.

The third compulsion comes later. Eventually, after sufficient cocaine, everyone acquires a paranoid mode of thinking. Some go on to hallucinate and become deluded. Upon recovery from the cocaine psychosis, a moderate or severe, occasionally suicidal, depression sets in. And the cure, transient though it be, is more cocaine.

The fourth urge to return to cocaine despite what has become a distinctly unpleasant existence is the anhedonia, the inability to feel that intervenes during the cocaine-free periods. What was once enjoyable is no longer so. Nothing is fun. The threshold of the reward or pleasure centers in the midbrain has been reset too high to make the ordinarily enjoyable aspects of life gratifying. In the end the only possible enjoyments are from cocaine.

The paradoxical situation in which consistent cocaine users finally find themselves—what started out as great fun winds up as a flight from dysphoria, anhedonia, and depression—is reflected in the frequency of relapse during efforts at treatment. An escape from the dulled discomfort back to the remembered bright peaks of cocaine euphoria is often irresistible.

How will the cocaine story end? Although it flies in the face of the present cocaine boom, I predict that it, too, will pass. This prediction is made on the basis of two experiences we have had with the powerful psychostimulants. One, just a century ago, was a 20-year-old love affair with cocaine. The wildly exaggerated statements heard then were even greater than the hyperbole emanating today from those in Stage I of cocaine use. It was not only the greatest lift, but it cured everything: alcoholism, morphine dependency, pain, depression, and even the common cold (See: *The New York Times* dated Sept. 2, 1885). It all fell apart in the late 1880s after too many became psychotic, overdosed, or disorganized from incessant cocaine use.

The second disaster with stimulants was the "speedfreak" spasm of a dozen years ago that looked like a sure winner for a while, but died after five short years. It consisted of the intravenous instillation of enormous amounts of methamphetamine and other amphetamines. It has been amply demonstrated that experienced users of the stimulants are unable to distinguish injected cocaine from equivalent amounts of amphetamines except that the latter drug lasts longer.

Why stimulant outbreaks have so little staying power is difficult to say. Perhaps they are too much. Speed may not always kill, but it does befuddle, disorganize, and deplete the consumer so that one can hardly go on. It is for such reasons that I would guess that the second coming of cocaine will subside. That does not mean that it will not return again someday after we have forgotten the story once more.

A FUTURIST'S VIEW OF ALCOHOL

What does the future hold for alcohol? Although it was originally a tribal social enhancer, tranquilizer, analgesic, and anesthetic, it has succeeded exceedingly well in adapting to modern, urban settings. It still serves many personal and group functions, still is sought after to diminish the cares of the day, and to achieve intoxication by those who prefer that state to sobriety.

All classes and races are involved with fermented or distilled beverages, so it comes close to being the universal solvent for human cares. Poverty is no bar, in fact, the poorest are among the most afflicted. Neither does affluence protect in any way from destructive drinking styles. It has displaced the indigenous intoxicants used by remote tribes and has more than held its own against the recent surges of cannabis and other drug use. Although a generally cited statistic is that one in ten drinkers becomes disabled in some way, the fact that nine of ten remain unimpaired tells us that disability is unnecessary when restraint is practiced. It is quite impossible to discern an end to humanity's involvement with ethanol.

Assuming that this civilization will continue to become increasingly complex and interlocking, what will be the future role of alcoholic beverages? As increasing demands are made upon people for alertness, precision, and complex mentation, will alcohol consumption be too dulling and disruptive to be permitted? Even now flight crews, air controllers, radar operators, and other job holders in sensitive positions are forbidden to consume alcohol up to 24 hours before going on duty. In other industries where complicated psychomotor skills are needed, using intoxicating substances coming to work or while at work are grounds for dismissal. Today the price we pay for overdrinking is too much. Tomorrow the price will be higher.

Nevertheless, there is no reason to believe that beverage alcohol will be prohibited or become obsolete in the coming centuries. It is not only deeply ingrained in the cultural matrix, but it is also a cost-efficient (but far from ideal) relaxant, disinhibitor, and social lubricant. It helps people deal with the harsh scrape of reality, and in the world of tomorrow, existence may be harsh, indeed. If high technology societies produce increasing impersonality and dehumanization, alcohol may be in greater demand than ever.

Admittedly, the aggressive and destructive behaviors evoked by alcohol will have to be much better controlled than they are at present. Solutions for disrupting undesired conduct can be found. For example, breathometers placed where alcohol is dispensed and installing them into the ignition system of vehicles may be helpful in avoiding a small part of the destruction. Increased leisure time will serve to intensify the demand for alcohol or something like it well into the future. Of course, if our scientists could somehow develop a maturation potion, then we might become a species of moderate drinkers. But such a scenario is based more on fantasy than on a realistic estimate of what will be.

WHAT ABOUT NARCOTICS?

Although heroinism in this country has remained relatively stable for the past few years or even declined, there is no reason to believe that the end of the opiate addiction is in sight. What has happened is that a world-wide shift in the distribution of heroin addiction has taken place. It has increased enormously in countries like Burma and Thailand and to a lesser degree in Western Europe and other countries where heroin dependence hardly existed in the past. So the problem is not going away; it is developing a wider world base.

It is possible that with the advent of the endogenous opioid peptides and the narcotic agonist-antagonists that are arriving on the marketplace, the need to prescribe addictive narcotics will diminish. Perhaps the requirement to grow opium crops will become superfluous. If one day every oriental poppy should disappear from the earth would that necessarily mean the end of narcotic addiction? I am afraid not. It is technically possible to synthesize narcotics that are many times more potent than heroin. The drug syndicates have the biochemists and the production specialists who are capable of manufacturing synthetic opiates, if necessary, in sufficient amounts to sustain the narcotic traffic. The supply control battlefield may drift from the opium plantation to the mobile laboratory.

Continuing breakdowns in familial and national cohesiveness along with increased social dissonance can lead to a resurgent interest in opiate usage. On the other hand, an increase in authoritarian governments could reduce the possibility that its members will have access to efficiency-reducing drugs. Admittedly, totalitarian regimes have not been completely successful in deterring their citizens from drunkenness, perhaps because of their own inefficiency. The future of opiate addiction can hardly be predicted at this time because of the multiple conflicting variables that may intervene.

SUMMARY

The outlook over time is mixed. Some mood-altering agents will fade away, others will persist, even grow. The nature of future societies will shape the need for and the ability to control chemicals that can cause behavioral problems.

The new world is difficult to assess. It may be the most humanizing or the most dehumanizing of places. As we change with our new environment, so will our use of drugs for the mind.

47. Paraphernalia

One spinoff of the multibillion-dollar drug abuse industry is the billion-dollar paraphernalia business. It is not quite enough these days to smoke pot rolled in cigarette paper; now the paper must be double width, scented, flavored, and embossed.

Cocaine is hardly ever inhaled through an ordinary straw; gold and silver tooters are being employed instead. Thousands of stores across the country are selling drug accessories exclusively, or they are kept as a sideline in some record shops, novelty gift stores, or boutiques.

THEY CALL IT RECREATION

Paraphernalia has come to mean those items made to prepare, package, store, or use the so-called recreational drugs. The recreational drugs involved are usually marijuana and cocaine, but nitrous oxide, amyl and butyl nitrite, the hallucinogens, and sometimes opium are included under this rubric. Drugs like heroin, barbiturates, and amphetamines have been excluded at present, and the injection of all chemicals is not considered "in" by the better class "dopers."

WHY PARAPHERNALIA?

Items of paraphernalia are available that have no direct connection to actual drug use. Drug-oriented jewelry, T-shirts, or comic books are the peripheral fun and game items to be found in these establishments. Nearby, records with some drug theme, popular drug-oriented magazines, or other sources of misinformation may be displaced to facilitate better living through chemistry. These oddities can be considered accessories before the fact.

Most head shops will deal in items that assist or simplify the process of using one of the mind-altering drugs. The extrawide rolling papers and modern cigarette-rolling machines make it easier to prepare marijuana to be smoked.

Bongs are devices that concentrate the smoke, permitting the user to inhale a large quantity, thus producing a higher high. They are sometimes carbureted so that the smoke is forced into the mouth under pressure. Roach clips hold the last tiny butt of the marijuana joint for its ultimate consumption. Cocaine spoons, jewelled or made of precious metals, measure out the quantity to be snorted.

Some items are intended to enhance the effects of a drug. Freebase kits convert street cocaine hydrochloride to cocaine alkaloid, intensifying its effects when smoked. Isomerizers are alleged to convert THC acid into THC despite the fact that combustion in a cigarette or pipe will do the same thing at no cost.

Some head shops sell the legal mind-altering drugs like isobutyl nitrite (with lurid trade names such as Rush, Toilet Water, Locker Room, and Joc Aroma), or nitrous oxide cartridges normally used for whipping cream. Procaine, a mild euphoriant supposed to be a sort of beginner's cocaine, is also available in some shops. Spores for growing psilocybe mushrooms and poppy seeds, along with fertilizers and lamps to grow one's own opium, can be found in a few stores. A variety of dubious herbs, spices, and teas of variable activity ranging from none to mild are also part of the stock in trade. In addition to these, pseudodrugs like practice grass made of alfalfa are stocked for the young novice to train on before moving on to the real thing.

Stash containers designed to hide or protect their contents have been designed with some measure of ingenuity. Cans that looked like Coca-Cola were once used for this purpose until the company took the stash can manufacturer to court. Cans of soup and other innocent products have been modified to provide a compartment for concealing drugs. Scented candles, incenses, and aerosol sprays are available to mask the pungent odor of marijuana. A shelf of books is displayed, informing the reader how to smuggle drugs into the country, or alternatively, how to concoct a variety of psychochemicals.

Even the adulterants to cut the pure drugs can be obtained in paraphernalia stores. Items like lactose and mannitol, commonly used to dilute cocaine, are sold, but it is dealers rather than consumers who would be the likely market for these items. Test kits to check the melting point of the cocaine buy also are available as a means of determining how markedly the material has been adulterated. It works both ways: not only are the adulterants sold, but kits to remove the adulterants are also obtainable.

For the most paranoid customers, antibugging devices, money belts, and safes can be purchased. In some establishments fake ID cards and passports are available to those in need of them.

Despite the youthfulness of the clientele, sexual aids and other porno shop items are on sale. There is no end to the ingenuity of the euphoria purveyors. Even a small nasal irrigator, supposedly to reduce the irritant effects of cocaine, can be found next to the coke snorters.

WHAT DOES IT ALL MEAN?

The rapid development and spread of shops that sell accessories for use with mood-altering drugs reflect not only the widespread use of these substances, but also the need to smoke, snort, and swallow these euphoriants in style. A certain glamorization and snob appeal is evident in addition to whatever practical usefulness some of the paraphernalia provides.

The provocative antiestablishment nature of the trade is obvious. This is a time when many of the established values and standards are being questioned. A faddish quality to all this also is evident. It may be fashionable in some circles to wear a gold coke spoon on a necklace, but when the junior high school crowd starts wearing gold plated ones, something new and different will have to be designed for the swinging set. It also means that despite the cost of euphoriant drugs, money for these superfluous oddities is not lacking. We remain an affluent, if not an effluent, society.

Perhaps the greatest objection to the head shops is the aura of legitimacy they give to illegal drug use—especially to juveniles. Certainly, if the wherewithall to use the so-called recreational drugs is offered at the local shopping center, what can be wrong with doing hash, cocaine, and the rest? Not only do such places provide symbolic permission to engage in chemical dabbling, but they deliberately entice the younger age group with pipes designed as space guns, frisbees, and other juvenile equipment designed for smoking marijuana. T-shirts for "tots who toke" and a variety of other unamusing items belie the ostensible declaration that these enterprises do not serve minors.

THE COMMUNITY REACTION

The offensive aspects of the paraphernalia establishments have given rise to a remarkable counteroffensive. For the first time since the flood of hedonistic drug taking was unleashed, many community groups have arisen to oppose drug usage by children. They have taken direct aim at the head shops as the most visible target of their frustrations.

The reasons for the upsurge in community action are not difficult to identify. Parents are shaken up when their junior high school offspring are found to be "doing" pot, rush, or downers. They discover that many kids in the neighborhood are stoned part or all of their waking day. At least one member of the community becomes angry enough to organize the neighborhood.

Another reason for the strong public reaction which turns out to be more effective than most government programs, is the number of drug-related deaths or serious injuries involving young people. Statistics on this point hardly exist, but the increasing demand for expert witnesses in felony cases is becoming a subspecialty for many psychopharmacologists.

The number of two-paragraph notices on the back pages of newspapers about drug-related homicides and accidental deaths are impressive evidence. Single-car accidents in which the young driver is found to have drugs, with or without alcohol, in his bloodstream are on the increase. Young dealers are shot or knifed for their drug supplies or their cash. Overdose deaths, usually from some drug combination, are not decreasing. Accidental death to oneself or others while intoxicated, suicides, or homicides while under the influence all continue to occupy the courts and the coroners offices. When a loved child is lost in some senseless drug-connected manner, many parents feel compelled to do something about it.

Add to these tragedies the high visibility of paraphernalia stores, and it is easy to see why parent groups have organized to somehow influence the situation. Their lobbying for antiparaphernalia laws, and their exerting direct pressure on the owners and landlords of head shops is only one of many activities. They attempt to educate themselves and their children about the drugs involved. They have become much less permissive about their offsprings' behavior, and more restrictive about their unsupervised free time.

Determined efforts are made to clean up the school and its environs with the cooperation of the principal and teachers. Other community groups are being enlisted in the antidrug effort. The consciousness of everyone must be raised about the preadolescents' predicament—their having to make drug-using decisions at an early age—for prevention activities to be successful. All of the parents in a neighborhood must retrieve and reassume their responsibilities for their children, otherwise the youngsters will win the "but all my friends are doing it" game.

The success of such parent group efforts cannot be accurately measured at this time. It will take years before a reversal of adolescent drug taking can be accurately estimated. Still, certain small gains have been achieved. Some youngsters now have the courage to say "No" to their peers. Some parents have reviewed their priorities and spend more time with their children. A few have even decided to avoid smoking and drinking at home in order to provide a drug-free environment. Cigarette papers and popular drug-oriented publications have been removed from a number of convenience and drug stores. The head shops are now claiming they will not sell to underage youngsters. Certain items, clearly intended for children, have disappeared from view.

THE LEGAL QUESTION

Some merchandise, used with abused drugs, is quite legal. Small spoons, safety blades, cigarette paper, pipes, straws, etc., can hardly be barred from the marketplace because they happen to be used for socially unpopular practices. Advertising them is probably protected by the First Amendment. They cannot be seized without due process under the Fourth Amendment. Therefore, the first efforts of city and state ordinances usually were declared unconstitutional because of vague or improper language.

It is legally possible to regulate and license drug paraphernalia shops. They can be barred from areas near schools, churches, libraries, etc. Specific advertising restrictions may withstand First Amendment arguments. Ordinances forbidding the sale or gift of these materials to minors have been upheld. States have been successful in seizing and destroying drug accessories without arresting the possessor.

The Department of Justice and Drug Enforcement Administration have prepared a model federal antiparaphernalia act which can be adapted to the needs of states and municipalities. Not all sections have been court tested, but they have been adopted by a number of jurisdictions that want to do something about the paraphernalia outlets.

The Select Committee on Narcotics Abuse and Control, Lester Wolf, Chairman, held hearings on the paraphernalia issue on November 1, 1979. It recommended state, local, and possibly federal legislation regulating the sale and advertising of these items. During the hearings witnesses for the paraphernalia industry stated that about 150,000 people with an earning power of a billion dollars would be put out of work if the industry were abolished. This sort of argument seemed unimpressive to those present for it could also be used to justify protecting the Mafia and related operations from prosecution.

THE PARAPHERNALIA INDUSTRY RESPONSE

With the growth of community-generated opposition and of local legislation, paraphernalia manufacturers and dealers have found it necessary to organize. An Accessories Trade Association with regional branches and appropriate industry publications such as the Accessories Digest, have retained legal defense groups that will advise or defend their membership in court cases.

For the past two years the paraphernalia business has slowed down. Whether this is due to grassroots pressures, law enforcement, or the recession is difficult to say. Nevertheless, in many cities the paraphernalia outlet has become as familiar as porno shops, adult movies, and topless bars. It is believed that nationwide, between 15,000 and 25,000 retail stores sell drug accessories.

They make efforts to display their wares at respectable related conventions, to use the word "accessories" in preference to "paraphernalia," to invoke free enterprise in lobbying against antiparaphernalia laws, and to be more discreet in their advertising—all in the hope of gaining greater acceptance and avoiding harassment by citizen groups.

BIBLIOGRAPHY

- *Community and Legal Responses to Drug Paraphernalia.* Services Research Report, NIDA, DHEW Publication No. (ADM) 80-963, 1980.
- *Drug Paraphernalia.* Hearing before the Select Committee on Narcotics Abuse and Control. House of Representatives. U.S. Government Printing Office, Washington, D.C. 1980.

48. AIDS

What may be a new biologic phenomenon has been reported during the past three years. This is the acquired immune deficiency syndrome (AIDS), a condition in which the immune defenses of the body are markedly lowered. The syndrome is of interest to those concerned about drug abuse because almost 20 percent of all cases have been reported in intravenous illicit drug users. Some 6,000 patients have been admitted to hospitals in the United States. The mortality rate is approximately 50 to 75 percent. About 125 patients are mentioned in the literature from other countries. Just under half of the known cases in the United States have been seen in New York City, and about 20 percent of the patients are in California. One or two new cases are reported to the New York City Health Department each day.

WHICH GROUPS ARE AT RISK?

Homosexual or bisexual males with promiscuous sexual lifestyles constitute 71 percent of those afflicted. Instances of the syndrome in female homosexuals are not recorded. Intravenous drug abusers of both sexes are known, constituting 15 percent of the involved men and 53 percent of the involved women. Haitians of both sexes make up about 5 percent of all cases, or about 100 individuals. Less than 1 percent of the AIDS cases occur in hemophiliacs. These patients, of course, are all males, and they receive a factor from plasma for their bleeding episodes. A small residual group remains who belong to none of the above categories or for whom the risk factor is unknown. Males of all races between the ages of 24 to 45 account for more than 90 percent of the cases.

WHAT IS THE CAUSE AND THE NATURE OF AIDS?

The cause of AIDS is a human T-cell leukemia virus (HTLV III). It affects T-cell production, impairing cell-mediated immunity. It results in an inability of the body to defend itself against certain ordinarily harmless infections and tumors. These infections and tumors are called "opportunistic" because, while ordinarily not pathogenic, they become so in people with AIDS.

WHAT OPPORTUNISTIC DISORDERS
AFFECT AIDS PATIENTS?

A large number of bacterial, fungal, or viral infections of minimal virulence are possible disease producers. However, two diseases are generally associated with AIDS. One is Kaposi's sarcoma, a skin tumor of low-grade malignancy usually caused by a cytomegalic virus. It was described over a century ago in debilitated old men and in people with lymphomas. When it occurs in connection with AIDS, it is aggressive, invasive, and often fatal.

A protozoan, *Pneumocystis carinii*, produces a pneumonitis in most AIDS patients. It was known as a rare disease afflicting those with severe underlying disorders like leukemia and patients on immunosuppressive therapy used to prevent rejection of an organ transplant. A few people receiving high dose courses of cancer chemotherapy or whole body irradiation with considerable bone marrow suppression might also be subject to *Pneumocystis carinii* pneumonia. In AIDS patients this condition is extremely serious.

Sometimes, both Kaposi sarcoma and *Pneumocystis carinii* pneumonia are found in the same patient. Other opportunistic infections may develop with or without the two conditions mentioned above.

DOES NORMAL IMMUNITY RETURN
TO SUCCESSFULLY TREATED AIDS PATIENTS?

It does not appear that the immune system recuperates following recovery from the pneumonia. The AIDS patients are at risk of acquiring other opportunistic infections for an indefinite period.

WHEN DID AIDS FIRST BECOME
CLINICALLY APPARENT?

During 1979, tumor registries noticed an increase in the incidence of Kaposi sarcoma in young men. At about the same time, cases of pneumonitis due to *Pneumocystis carinii* began to show up in New York City hospitals.

HOW IS AIDS TRANSMITTED?

Direct contact with infected blood, feces, or semen seems necessary for transmission. It has similarities to viral hepatitis in this respect. Precautions ordinarily used with viral hepatitis patients should be taken by health care personnel.

WHAT ARE THE RISKS FOR PEOPLE IN CONTACT WITH A PERSON WITH AIDS?

It appears that intimate, direct encounters such as sexual contacts, or the injection of blood or blood products is necessary to transmit AIDS. Casual contacts with people in the incubation or active phases of the disease are not hazardous.

WHAT IS THE INCUBATION PERIOD?

The incubation period is long, probably from six months to three years or more. In a New York State correctional facility study, seven patients developed symptoms during incarceration. All had been intravenous narcotic or narcotic and cocaine users previous to their confinement. The average duration of imprisonment before diagnosis of *Pneumocystis carinii* pneumonia was 18.1 months, with a range of 5 to 38 months. None of these individuals were homosexual, nor had they had homosexual contacts in prison. They had used drugs intravenously for an average of 12 years previous to their sentencing.

The significance of the prolonged incubation period is that transmission of AIDS from healthy or slightly ill people becomes possible.

WHAT ARE THE PRODROMAL SYMPTOMS?

During the long, prodromal period a variety of nondescript complaints may be noted. Discomfort, unexplained weakness, and weight loss can occur early. Enlarged lymph nodes which, when biopsied, show nonspecific hyperplastic changes are not uncommon. Diarrheal episodes appear and subside. A leucopenia, particularly a lymphopenia, may be present. Cytomegalovirus and hepatitis infections can be found when laboratory studies are done.

WHAT ARE THE SYMPTOMS OF THE PNEUMONIA?

The *Pneumocystis carinii* penumonia begins with an unproductive cough, fatigue, and shortness of breath. Chills and fever, with temperatures up to 40° centigrade may be noted. Oral candidiasis (thrush) is often present. Complete blood counts show a mild anemia and a leucopenia with white counts varying from 2,000 to 5,000 cells/mm.[3] In a few instances the total white count has been higher. The leucopenia is predominantly due to a marked decrease in lymphocytes. Lymphocyte subtyping reveals decreased T-lymphocytes with the most marked reduction in T-helper cells. Chest X-rays reveal unilateral, but more typically, bilateral infiltrates. A lung biopsy may be necessary to establish the diagnosis of *Pneumocystis carinii* pneumonia.

HOW DOES THE KAPOSI SARCOMA PRESENT?

Kaposi tumors are multifocal, small, elevated, reddish blue or brown skin lesions. They may metastasize, extend to the regional lymph nodes, or appear on mucous membranes and the viscera. They are soft nodules and might be first seen on the extremities or trunk. They bleed when traumatized.

WHAT ARE THE SPECIAL FEATURES OF THE ADDICT WHO DEVELOPS AIDS?

The most frequent association with AIDS occurs in the intravenous drug user who shares needles with others. It does not matter which drug is injected. Intravenous cocaine and heroin users have developed AIDS. It is likely that any other drug administered in an unsterile fashion could transmit AIDS. The great majority of cases in addicts have occurred in the New York City metropolitan area.

One interesting, but unexplained, difference between the homosexual AIDS group and the intravenous drug AIDS group is the variation in clinical manifestations. In the homosexual cases about half have Kaposi sarcomas and most of the others have *Pneumocystis carinii* pneumonia with a small number having other opportunistic infections. The drug users develop Kaposi sarcomas about 10 percent of the time, get *Pneumocystis carinii* pneumonia in 70 percent of the cases, and present with other opportunistic infections in the remainder.

DO "POPPERS" HAVE ANYTHING TO DO WITH AIDS?

At one time a correlation between the volatile nitrites (amyl and butyl nitrites) and AIDS in patients seemed to indicate a causal relationship. It is now believed that since homosexual men are prone to develop AIDS, and since they use "poppers" as a sexual enhancer, the association is coincidental.

WHAT ABOUT OTHER DRUGS AND AIDS?

Marijuana is believed by some investigators to diminish immune responsivity through its effect upon the T-lymphocytes. Marijuana is frequently smoked by heroin users and male homosexuals. Investigations of the role of marijuana smoking indicate that its use is not a cause but an associated activity.

IS ANYTHING BEING DONE ABOUT AIDS?

More money will be spent on AIDS research in 1985 than was spent over an eight-year period on Legionnaire's Disease and toxic shock syndrome combined. This is happening, not only because AIDS is a deadly disease that could spread to other populations, but also because the basic nature of the immune process may be illuminated by understanding AIDS.

WHAT ABOUT TREATMENT?

Synthetic interferon, an antibody present in most mammalian species, is being tried. Results have not yet been published. The pneumonitis is treated with antibiotics like trimethoprim-sulfamethoxazole and pentamidine. The sarcoma cannot be treated with the usual cancer chemotherapeutic agents because they suppress the immune system. The antibiotics also reduce lymphocyte counts. It is predicted that a preventive vaccine will become available in a few years.

HOW ABOUT PREVENTION?

During the past three years AIDS has been increasing exponentially and spreading with geometric progression. Its containment is a concern of all people, and particularly of the vulnerable populations.

The use of needles to penetrate the skin removes a powerful barrier to AIDS and other infections. Those drug users who employ needles should rethink their mode of usage because of the new danger presented by AIDS. Sharing the "works" increases the risk. Ordinary sterilization methods may not be sufficient to destroy the AIDS factor. The fact that the majority of needle users come down with hepatitis B sooner or later means they do not use sterile techniques and are vulnerable to AIDS.

The male homosexual lifestyle often includes random promiscuity and unusual sexual practices that bring them into contact with blood, semen, feces, and other body fluids of their partners. AIDS demands that these activities be reconsidered.

There is a possibility that bisexual men could transmit the syndrome to heterosexual women. In that manner, the heterosexual community could become involved, although it is not established that nontraumatic genital sex can transmit AIDS.

SUMMARY

We are in the early stages of a novel and serious contagious disease that could subside spontaneously, but is just as likely to continue to spread unless countermeasures are found to bring it under control. We have good information on how it is disseminated, and correcting certain unphysiologic lifestyles could halt AIDS. Unfortunately, changing lifestyles of large numbers of individuals is difficult even under the threat of acquiring a fearsome disease.

49. Therapeutic Communities for Substance Abusers

The gathering of small numbers of like-minded, nonrelated people who have withdrawn from the dominant society and who have joined together for mutual aid has existed for millenia. In ancient times these clusters separated themselves for religious reasons. The Hebrew Essenes, the German Anabaptists, and the various monastic orders either could not tolerate or were persecuted by the prevailing religious practitioners. Others recognized the need for distance from an unacceptable existence and for a contemplative, devoted, and disciplined life style.

Susequently, retreats were formed based on political differences with the established system. The communes of seventeenth-century France and Gandhi's ashrams were examples of such grouping and hermitages. Many other groups have abandoned ordinary existence for spiritual or philosophic reasons. This banding together took place especially during times of decadence and turmoil.

Maxwell Jones is generally credited with the first formation of a therapeutic community (TC) for psychotherapeutic purposes. In 1958 the first TC, Synanon, was formed to provide a residential, nonmedical setting for the recovery from heroin addiction. It was founded by Chuck Dederich in Santa Monica, California and has served as a model for some 500 subsequent TCs in this country and abroad. Daytop Village, Gaudenzia House, Phoenix House, and Odyssey House are but a few of the derivative communities that adopted the Synanon experience.

OPERATIONAL BASIS FOR TCs

In order to understand whatever successes the TCs have had, it must be recognized that attitude and behavior changes are readily accomplished when an individual's access to information is completely controlled. This shaping of attitudes and behavior is well known to those involved in brainwashing activities, boot camps, political indoctrination, and cult programming. In addition, TCs have employed a number of other techniques in an effort to alter the addicts' immature and inappropriate responses to life. Not every TC utilizes all of the items mentioned below, but some are discernible in every TC.

1. An *arduous admission policy* eliminates those with low levels of motivation and makes acceptance into the TC a valued accomplishment. More recently, acceptance into many TCs has become much less selective.

2. *Charismatic leadership* is notable at Synanon and other TCs. An omnipotent, authoritarian figure can take over all decision-making requirements.

3. The primacy of *personal responsibility* for one's own rehabilitation is emphasized.

4. *Mutual assistance.* An oft-cited TC quotation is: "You alone can do it, but you cannot do it alone." The assistance varies from straightening the resident out in an encounter group to supporting him or her during some difficult period.

5. *Self-examination and confession.* The resident is urged to examine himself or herself with the help of other members and then confess to stupidities and childishness in their presence.

6. The need for *structure and discipline* in the addict's life is obvious. In a TC every hour of the day is accounted for, and one's behavior is under constant scrutiny.

7. *Rewards and punishments* are meted out according to the appropriateness or inappropriateness of the behavior involved. Learning through positive and negative reinforcement is a fundamental aspect of TC manipulation. Rising in the hierarchy or obtaining certain privileges are examples of rewards. Common punishments are the "haircut," actually shaving the head, or putting the individual in the "hot seat" of an encounter session.

8. The TC serves the functions of an *extended family* or tribal collective.

9. The TC resident is initially *separated from society*. The separation gives the resident an interval away from drugs, friends, and family, a milieu in which he or she had failed in the past. This break in continuity permits a sort of psychological rebirth or, at least, a new beginning. The TC is also more or less distanced from society in order to better control the member's behavior. In the early days opposition by the power structure provided cohesiveness and intensified bonding within the TC.

10. Early in the development of TCs there were *no authority figures* except for the leader. Staff functioned on the same level as residents. More recently, professionals have come into the TC, and they serve in authority roles.

11. Attitudes of nonviolence, self-reliance, honesty, and responsibility are fostered. The nonviolence is physical—verbal violence is permitted, even encouraged. These goals are the same as those professed by the "square" world outside. Many other similarities between TC values and idealistic capitalism exist, including:

12. *Emphasis on work.* Everybody works. They contribute to the maintenance of the facility, they learn proper work habits, and they acquire new job skills. Work is a part of therapy in TCs.

TC POLICIES

If the resident required detoxification from heroin, "cold turkey" was prescribed. He or she was literally given a bed and a bucket—and community support. At present detoxification is accomplished under medical supervision. Methadone may be used for detoxification, but drug abstinence is the rule thereafter.

The length of a residential stay varies from three months to a lifetime depending on the TC. Whether sufficient psychological maturation can be accomplished in a few months has been questioned. Synanon believes that the outside world is corrupt and unlivable, and reentry into it is not a proper goal.

The optimal size of a TC is about 50 people. When it becomes too large, it divides into two TCs. Groups smaller than 25 tend not to be cost effective.

Residents start at the bottom (often by cleaning the toilet bowls.) They work their way up to the top echelon. Discharge planning begins well before the expected date, and the resident is given increasing time to spend on passes, or he or she is sent to a halfway house to look for a job and to diminish the culture shock of reentry.

PROBLEMS CONFRONTING TCs

A number of perennial problems that confront TCs have remained unresolved or only partially solved. They will be briefly discussed.

1. *The closed information system.* Mention has already been made of the advantages of controlling information input to produce attitudinal change.

However, it also poses problems. Restricting communications from outside permits closed loop messages to reverberate uncritically among group members. This can lead to a situation in which arbitrary and unwise decisions are allowed to prevail. At Synanon, marital dissolutions and vasectomies for all were ordained. The Wire, a system of transmitting the Founder's message to evey Synanon member, was installed. It provided guidance on matters large and small. Eventually, an armed military unit was formed to protect the TC from hostile outsiders. Their activities culminated in an attempted murder.

2. *Sexuality*. How to foster group closeness without encouraging sexual acting out has been a concern of many TCs. Resident-resident and staff-resident sexual alliances are permitted in some TCs and interdicted in others.

3. *Drinking and "soft" drug use*. Whether alcohol and marijuana are permissible has usually been decided by insisting on abstinence. Synanon has forbidden tobacco.

4. *Ethnic and gender differences*. The different needs of women and those of minority cultural backgrounds were hardly considered until recently. Many TCs have modified their practices to accommodate these groups' special requirements.

5. *Staff disunity*. Serious differences between clinical and administrative staff and between paraprofessionals and professionals continue to emerge. Paraprofessionals are almost invariably recovered addicts who have excellent "street" knowledge, but the professionals have acquired the background and education to provide counseling. Rivalries exist despite the fact that both have much to learn from each other. The conflict has not diminished with the movement of TCs toward the conventional health care framework.

6. *Funding*. This has been a perennial source of concern. Hope of becoming eligible for third-party payments has accelerated licensing and accreditation efforts. Problems remain.

7. *Staff burnout*. Staff loss of effectiveness and accelerated turnover is a continuing problem. All types of drug treatment facilities share this problem with the TCs.

8. *The polydrug abuser*. Traditionally, the TC client was the heroin-dependent person. The polydrug abuser is becoming at least as numerous. They are quite different demographically and, perhaps, characterologically. The TCs have had to try to adapt to the special needs of managing the polydrug abuser.

9. *The split rate*. An unacceptably high split rate has plagued the TC movement. Dropouts are understandable since a considerable degree of motivation is required to stay until graduation. More than three-quarters of those who enter will leave before completion of the program. Therefore, the results are poor if everyone is counted. They are excellent if only graduates are counted.

FUTURE DIRECTIONS

The TCs are changing in an effort to meet new challenges. The trend seems to include linkages with established health services. This may resolve the conflict between the desire to be independent of the system versus the need for a stable source of support. The paraprofessionals will inevitably become professionalized, providing improved counseling skills, job security, and vertical and horizontal mobility. In order to justify continuing support of the TCs a system of evaluation and accountability will be required to measure outcome and cost effectiveness.

SUMMARY

TCs have provided the substance abuse field with some outstanding leaders. They will continue to play a significant role in the management of selected drug-dependent people. Their contribution, though, is a partial one with only about 10 percent of all drug-dependent people willing to enter such programs, or if they do, willing to remain in the program.

BIBLIOGRAPHY

- Brook, R.C. and Whitehead, P.C. *Drug Free Therapeutic Community.* Human Sciences Press, New York, 1980.
- Deitch, D.A. and Zweben, J.E. Synanon: A pioneering response to drug abuse treatment and a signal for caution. In: *Substance Abuse: Clinical Problems and Perspectives.* Eds.: Lowinson, J.H. & Ruiz, P. Williams & Wilkins, Baltimore, 1981, pp. 289-302.
- DeLeon, G. and Andrews, M. Therapeutic community dropouts 5 years later: Preliminary findings on self reported status. In: *A Multicultural View of Drug Abuse.* Eds.: D.E. Smith et al., G.K. Hall/Schenkman, Cambridge, MA., 1978, pp. 369-377.
- DeLeon, G. and Rosenthal, M.S. Therapeutic Communities. In: *Hand-*

book on Drug Abuse. Eds.: R.I. Dupont, A. Goldstein & J. O'Donnell, U.S. Government Printing Office, Washington, D.C. 20402, 1979, pp. 39-47.

- O'Brien, W.B. and Biase, D.V. The therapeutic community: The family-milieu approach to recovery. In: *Substance Abuse: Clinical Problems and Perspectives*. Eds.: Lowinson, J.H. & Ruiz, P. Williams & Wilkins, Baltimore, 1981, pp. 303-316.

50. Opiates and Endorphins for Mental Illness

SCHIZOPHRENIA

A fairly common clinical observation is that certain chronic schizophrenics have a reduced perception of pain. Two personal observations are particularly vivid. One is of a chronic schizophrenic patient who looked ill, but who had no complaints except tiredness. A few days later, he fainted, went into shock, and died. At post-mortem he had coronary thrombosis of the left main artery and a large myocardial infarction.

A second incident was the observation of an alert psychiatric aide who reported a urinal had red stains that could have been blood. By doing urine analyses of the entire ward, a chronic psychiatric patient with hematuria was identified before the specimen was sent to the laboratory. He was found to have an urethral calculus in transit and should have been in great pain from renal colic. Neither of these patients was mute or totally withdrawn. Others who have worked with chronic schizophrenics can duplicate such stories.

In one study, about one-third of chronic schizophrenics did not present with signs of, or complain of pain from, acute perforated peptic ulcers, acute appendicitis, or femoral fractures. A majority of psychotic patients who were later found to have myocardial infarctions also did not complain of pain.

In earlier days such analgesia to what would ordinarily be a painful injury or illness was thought to be owing to the preoccupation of psychotics with delusions. Alternatively they were considered to be in a permanently stressful internal state and that stress-induced analgesia existed.

In the light of the recent discoveries of internal opiate-like peptides and of specific opioid bindings sites, the hypoalgesia or analgesia might be reconsidered as an overproduction of endorphins or enkephalins (hyperendorphinism?), or a change, perhaps a sensitization, of the opioid receptors. It has been speculated that distortions of endorphin activity might cause, be associated with, or be the result of the schizophrenic process. At this time no answers are at hand, but some of the research will be reviewed to reflect the current state of these matters.

Another line of clinical experience suggests a hypothesis that seems opposite to the one derived from some schizophrenics' diminished pain perception. In preneuroleptic days narcotics were used to treat psychotic states. Opium has long been employed to manage what is now called schizophrenia, and it reduced many symptoms of that disorder. Psychotic behavior, in particular, was contained.

A more recent observation is pertinent. It has been noted that when schizophrenic opiate addicts are detoxified, a few experience an exacerbation of their mental disease. When these patients are placed on methadone maintenance, they seem to have better control over their bizarre conduct. A few achieve better levels of functioning while on methadone than during neuroleptic therapy. Another observation: When patients on antipsychotic drugs are placed on methadone maintenance, a lower dose of their antipsychotic medication may be needed. Are these effects a result of the nonspecific sedative effects of opioids, or do they represent alterations in opioid receptor saturation, which in turn, has a dopamine-blocking activity?

Both opiates and endorphins have neuroleptic-like effects. Both diminish or block dopamine receptor cell activity, and both increase prolactin levels, a characteristic common to all active neuroleptics. Increased prolactin secretion is only a marker of diminished dopamine blockade at dopaminergic postsynaptic neurons in the limbic system. Dopamine blockade probably causes the antipsychotic action; prolactin elevation and other neuroendocrine changes are simply associated effects.

There are also differences between opioids and neuroleptics. Beta endorphin injected in rats' cerebral ventricles produces a rigid immobility (catatonia?) and a loss of the righting reflex followed by hyperactivity. The narcotic antagonist naloxone will reverse the immobility. In contrast, haloperidol administered similarly does not induce this picture.

As might be predicted, when schizophrenics are treated with endogenous or exogenous opioids, the results are variable and inconclusive. Schizophrenia is a syndrome that has many causes. It should not be expected that it will respond uniformly to treatment. One study that probably should be done is to select out pain-insensitive schizophrenics and expose them to a trial of narcotic agonists and antagonists like naloxone. They may constitute one schizophrenic subgroup that is more homogeneous than those investigated up to this time.

The schizophrenia/endorphin hypotheses have been sardonically characterized in the literature as follows:

1. There is a quantitative problem:
   a. too much endorphin,
   b. too little endorphin.

c

2. There is a qualitative problem:
   a. altered endorphin,
   b. altered endorphin ratios,
   c. altered receptors.

3. There is no endorphin problem:
   a. the explanation lies elsewhere,
   b. there is no explanation.

This listing pretty well covers the various possibilities. When an important discovery of knowledge comes forth, there is a blizzard of activity. We are now in the blizzard phase of opioid and opioid receptor research. The data have produced an almost impenetrable storm, and only a few dim outlines of the terrain are visible. A similar confusing flurry of activity occurred in the 1950s when ACTH and cortisone appeared on the scene. Eventually, the storm will subside, and we will be able to map the endorphin role with more precision. The final appraisal will not be a simple one.

DEPRESSION

Major depressions are said to be associated with an elevated or disturbed pain threshold and an increased pain tolerance. The information about pain perception in manics is incomplete, but they, too, may have hypoalgesia. These responses refer to somatic pain or experimental pain. That depressives may complain bitterly of pain is well known, but this represents either a depressive equivalent or a culturally acceptable way to describe psychic depression.

The elevated pain threshold in depressed patients is attributed to increased endorphin receptor activity. They will become hyperalgesic if naltrexone, a narcotic antagonist, is administered.

Opium and its alkaloids and related compounds have beed widely used as a treatment for melancholia. Eighty years ago Kraepelin praised tincture of opium for its antidepressant effect. More recently small numbers of people have been given short courses of beta endorphin, and they appeared to have decreased depressive symptomatology for a few hours. There is evidence that depressives are people under stress. They often have elevated cortisol levels, and the dexamethasone suppression test is used as a test for melancholia. It is interesting that both ACTH and beta endorphin are produced from beta lipoprotein in response to stress. The production of cortisol and beta endorphin may occur in response to external and internal stressors. Most clinical studies of depression have involved administering opioids while those in manic patients have used narcotic antagonists. In addition, mixed agonists-antagonists (buprenorphine) have been tried in depressive states. One researcher found that bipolar depressed patients given beta endorphin either were improved or became manic. The results have been mixed; that is, improvement, worsening, or no effects have been reported.

MISCELLANEOUS CONDITIONS

Insufficient evidence is present in the conditions noted below to be certain of the findings reported to date.

The subgroup of placebo responders is likely to show an increased level of opiate receptor binding in response to a placebo.

Acupuncture raises cerebrospinal fluid levels of methionine enkephalin, and acupuncture analgesia is reversed by naloxone.

Despite high hopes that the discoveries of internal opioids and their receptors would help improve the prevention or treatment of narcotic dependence, no breakthroughs can be reported. The hypothesis that three, possibly four, specific receptors can be discriminated does lend hope to the notion that the analgesic action of opioids can be divorced from their euphoriant effect. It has been found that during withdrawal from chronic opiate use, beta endorphins are increased in spinal fluid. This may represent nothing more than the already mentioned stress response with release of endogenous opioids. It is fairly well established that endorphins will abort the morphine withdrawal symptoms.

The internal opioids may play a role in the regulation of food intake. Beta endorphin stimulates food intake in satiated rats. Naloxone reduces eating in starved rats and it abolishes overeating in obese rodents.

Electroconvulsive treatments significantly increase beta endorphin levels. This also represents a stress response. Many psychiatric treatments during the dark ages of psychiatry may well have produced improvement because they were stress-inducing procedures like being whirled in a cage, being dipped in to cold water, and having one's colon removed. Indeed, endorphin activity is increased following major surgical procedures, and this has nothing to do with the anesthetic. Interestingly, the beta endorphin level found during surgery correlates inversely with the patients's morphine requirements in the postoperative period.

A small number of individuals have a congenital absence of pain sensation. This can be a serious condition since the warning function of pain is unavailable. A few of these people were found to have high beta endorphin levels in their cerebrospinal fluid. If this finding can be replicated, it suggests that narcotic antagonist treatment may be indicated.

SUMMARY

No other area of neuroscience research is as active as investigations of endorphins, enkephalins, and their longer-acting ligands. To highlight this intense endorphillia, the November 7, 1978, issue of *Science* appeared with the second *E* missing on its front page. The explanatory caption stated that due to a temporary shortage of *Es* caused by the large number of papers on endorphins and enkephalins, the final *E* had to be omitted. This bountiful harvest has continued and shows no signs of abating.

In attempting to review the vast literature and make sense of it results in stress-induced analgesia, one is numbed by the complexity of the problem and the contradictory reports. It may be that this confusion is part of the scientific method. When a major and exciting field opens, it naturally attracts many investigators. They are forced to use new and unstandardized substances, procedures, and methods. Over time, the tangled threads are slowly rearranged until the warp and woof transform into a meaningful pattern. That time is not yet here for the peptide narcotics. Their role in psychiatric illness remains obscure.

BIBLIOGRAPHY

In addition to a number of individual papers, the following collected articles were used in preparation of this essay:

- *Opioids in Mental Illness: Theories, Clinical Observations and Treatment Possibilities*. Karl Verebey, Ed., Annals N.Y. Acad. Sci. 398:1-510, 1982.
- *Opiate Receptors, Neurotransmitters and Drug Dependence: Basic Science - Clinical Correlates*. Barry Stimmel, Ed., Advances in Alcohol and Substance Abuse, 1:1-123, 1981, Haworth Press.

51. Clonidine (Catapres): Nonopiate Detoxification

Clonidine is a drug known to be effective in the management of some hypertensive patients. The mechanism of action is a central alpha adrenergic stimulation. This results in an *inhibition* of the sympathetic vascoconstrictor and cardioaccelerator centers in the medulla and a diminished sympathetic autonomic outflow from the brain. The heart is slowed, cardiac output is reduced, and the vasodilation of peripheral vessels all combine to reduce the arterial blood pressure.

One major site of action for the hypotensive effect of clonidine must be the locus ceruleus (the blue spot) situated at the floor of the fourth ventricle of the brain. This is an important shunting station for alpha-2-adrenergic activity. Undoubtedly, other psychophysiologic effects are generated here in addition to the dilation of blood vessels and the reduction in heart rate, since the locus ceruleus has important connections with not only the spinal sympathetic centers, but also the limbic system and the cerebral cortex. These appear to be important emotion-modulating activities involved in locus ceruleus inhibition.

It has been well established that opiates and endorphins reduce the firing of the alpha adrenergic neurons. This means that the opiate receptors must have the important task of influencing the brain's noradrenergic centers. When heroin or similar narcotics are taken to the point of dependence, not only is the release of endogenous opioid peptides inhibited, but the activity of the locus ceruleus is also inhibited.

If the use of the opiate is then suddenly stopped, a characteristic series of abstinence symptoms emerges. Typically, they may include lacrimation, diarrhea, chilliness, rhinorrhea, muscle and joint pains and jerks, stomach cramps, agitation, yawning, dilated pupils, nausea, hypertension, insomnia, fever, increased pulse and respiratory rates, and gooseflesh. Many of these symptoms are well correlated with peripheral sympathetic overactivity.

The narcotic withdrawal syndrome is not only unpleasant when large amounts of high quality narcotics have been taken for long periods of time, but it can be life-endangering for elderly or medically ill people. Therefore, it is customary to gradually reduce the narcotic dose (detoxification). The more strenuous cold turkey treatment (so-called because of the gooseflesh present) in which the patient is provided with nothing but "a bed and a bucket" is sometimes used under nonmedical conditions. The usual medical procedure consists of switching the patient to about 20 to 40 mg of oral methadone a day from the narcotic that he or she has been abusing. Then, the dose is reduced by about 5 mg a day, until the patient is made opiate-free in relative comfort. From 7 to 21 days are usually allowed for complete detoxification to take place.

Simply eliminating narcotics from the addict is not a treatment; it is only the beginning of treatment. As little as 1 to 5 percent of those who receive detoxification alone will remain abstinent thereafter.

The disadvantage of methadone detoxification is that methadone is a narcotic, and some patients, eager to get off all narcotics, are sometimes reluctant to take it. Furthermore, a large percentage of those being detoxified quit even before the brief weaning period is completed.

If heroin suppresses sympathetic autonomic activity and clonidine is an alpha-2 adrenergic agonist, then it seemed reasonable to Gold and Kleber to try clonidine for the heroin withdrawal syndrome since the symptoms resemble an enormous burst of sympathetic overactivity. It should be recalled that alpha adrenergic stimulation results in an inhibition of peripheral sympathetic discharge.

An advantage of a nonnarcotic type of detoxification would be that if narcotic antagonist treatment with naltrexone is planned, the necessary delay between detoxification with methadone and the onset of naltrexone treatment is eliminated. All opiates must be out of the system before a narcotic antagonist is given, else withdrawal symptoms will be precipitated.

A theoretical benefit that has not yet been studied is that maintaining the detoxified person on small doses of clonidine might avoid the protracted abstinence syndrome that appears to last for months and may be the cause of certain relapses. The protracted abstinence syndrome consists of subtle changes in autonomic function in former addicts given a dose of morphine long after detoxification.

CLINICAL STUDIES WITH CLONIDINE

In initial studies on a total of 23 individuals abruptly withdrawn from either heroin or methadone maintenance, clonidine appeared to produce a significant reduction in withdrawal symptoms. The heroin-using subjects had been addicted for 2 to 10 years, and the subjects on methadone maintenance had been taking methadone for 6 to 60 months. Prior to the administration of clonidine, these subjects were denied opiates for at least 36 hours and were experiencing withdrawal symptoms. In all subjects the administration of 5 micrograms of clonidine per kg twice a day was followed by a highly significant reduction of opiate withdrawal symptoms with the identical placebo showing negligible effects.

All of the patients who were offered the option of continuing to take clonidine 5 micrograms per kg per day chose clonidine over a return to methadone maintenance. After a week, clonidine was discontinued, and no withdrawal symptoms were observed even after a naloxone challenge. Later, a 14-day inpatient study was carried out on 30 methadone dependent patients. In this study a larger dose of clonidine, 17 micrograms per kg per day, for the first 10 days was used. The higher dose was chosen because close supervision was possible, and because the withdrawal from methadone is known to be more difficult than from other opiates. All the patients completed the study and were successfully detoxified.

In another study involving a total of 70 patients, two methods of clonidine detoxification were evaluated. One involved a gradual reduction of methadone with simultaneous administration of clonidine, and the other an abrupt switch from methadone and/or heroin to clonidine. The occurrence and severity of withdrawal symptoms were less in the rapid detoxification group than in the gradual withdrawal group, and the success rate was better than that reported for methadone detoxification.

Although these are early findings, the data look encouraging. It appears that increases in brain-noradrenergic functioning mediate most symptoms of opiate withdrawal. Perhaps much more will be learned about the nature of the entire process of dependence and of the interaction of opiate receptors with alpha adrenergic receptors.

ADVERSE EFFECTS OF CLONIDINE

Naturally, there are problems. While the clinical work on the use of clonidine in opiate withdrawal has been encouraging, the drug does possess properties that could limit its usefulness. In high doses, clonidine can cause severe hypotension, sluggishness, drowsiness, and dryness of the mouth.

Perhaps the most serious potential consequence of clonidine therapy is the possibility of a clonidine withdrawal syndrome upon discontinuation of the drug. The withdrawal syndrome is known in patients receiving clonidine for hypertension who abruptly discontinue the drug. It involves a rebound increase in blood pressure. It has been fatal in hypertensives. In the studies involving the treatment of opiate withdrawal, no evidence of clinically significant rebound hypertension occurred.

Apparently the duration of the clonidine administration used in these studies ranging from one to two weeks is insufficiently long to evoke the reactive hypertension. Nervousness, agitation, and headache are also part of the cloni-dine withdrawal syndrome. It would seem prudent to gradually reduce the clonidine dosage even for opiate detoxification.

Another limitation of clonidine therapy of opiate addiction is that not all symptoms of opiate dependence can be controlled with clonidine. In most in-stances opiate withdrawal symptoms have been satisfactorily reduced, but not completely eliminated by clonidine.

The Gold-Kleber group at Yale recently reported a provocative finding. In six patients who had been successfully detoxified with clonidine, episodes of anxiety, panic, and depression were subsequently observed. This observation supports the notion that for some patients, methadone maintenance does not simply help keep them off street opiates, but it also serves as a psychotropic therapy for their depression, psychosis, or panic states. If this is so, clonidine (or other detoxification measures) is not appropriate for such individuals un-less accompanied by antidepressants, antipsychotics, or anxiolytics. These data also give support to the long-held belief that opiates have some antide-pressant and antipanic activity.

SUMMARY

If it is substantiated that opiates produce a depression of sympathetic activ-ity and that the opiate withdrawal syndrome is essentially a rebound of height-ened sympathetic activity, valuable information will have been gained. The fact that clonidine, an alpha-2-adrenergic agonist, can control much of the symptomatology of narcotic withdrawal is an interesting theoretical and clin-ical piece of information.

The anatomical basis for much of clonidine's effects is the locus ceruleus. The reported instances of the exacerbation of emotional disturbances after detoxification with clonidine may open new insights about the role of the cen-tral adrenergic system in emotional illness. Finally, we can assume that a sub-group of opiate addicts uses these drugs in an effort at self-treatment of under-lying emotional disturbances.

BIBLIOGRAPHY

- Gold, M.S., Redmond, D.E. and Kleber, H.D. Clonidine Blocks Acute Opiate Withdrawal Symptoms. *Lancet.* 1:929-930, 1978.
- Gold, M.S. and Kleber, H.D. "A Rationale for Opiate Withdrawal Symptomology." *Drug and Alcohol Dependence*, 4, 419-424, 1979.
- Gold, M.S., Potlash, A.L.C., Sweeney, D.R., Kleber, H.D. and Red-mond, D.E. Rapid Opiate Detoxification: Clinical Evidence of Antide-

pressant and Antipanic Effects of Opiates. *American Journal of Psychiatry*, 136: 982, 1979.

● Gold, M.S., Redmond, D.E. and Kleber, H.D. Noradrenergic Hyperactivity in Opiate Withdrawal Supported by Clonidine Reversal of Opiate Withdrawal. *American Journal of Psychiatry*, 136: 100, 1979.

● Washton, A.M., Resnick, R.B. and Rawson, R.A. Clonidine Hydrochloride: A Nonopiate Treatment for Opiate Withdrawal. In: *Problems of Drug Dependence, 1979*, L.S. Harris, Ed., NIDA Research Monograph #27, 1979.

● Kosman, M.E. Evaluation of Clonidine Hydrochloride (Catapress): A New Antihypertensive Agent, *JAMA*. 233: 174, 1975.

52. The Chronic Intractable Benign Pain Syndrome

The rational management of acute and acute, recurrent pain remains less than optimal. The treatment of chronic pain is a more difficult problem and is much less effectively handled. In this essay, one type of chronic pain, the chronic intractable benign pain syndrome (CIBPS), will be discussed. Other forms of consistent pain, like the pain that sometimes accompanies terminal cancer, central pain (tic douloureux, postherpetic neuralgia, phantom limb pain, etc.) will not be covered.

DEFINITION OF THE SYNDROME

This quite common condition is called "benign" only insofar as it is not associated with a malignant tumor. Its course is often far from benign. CIBPS is usually not related to a pathologic or pathophysiologic process, although trauma may have precipitated the original complaints. The location is usually the low back, or neck, or both. Certain types of headaches can be included in CIBPS. The DSM III diagnosis of psychogenic pain disorder approximates the CIBPS.

Because of a long-standing preoccupation with pain and suffering, the patient's psychosocial functioning is seriously disturbed in a number of ways. A dysphoric mood or a full-blown depression is evident. Hysterical or hypochondriacal personality features may be present. Many of the CIBPS patients are dependent on narcotics or sedatives, and tolerance to these drugs increases their drug-seeking behavior. In addition, they may be experiencing some of the side effects of these depressant medications: oversedation or intoxication. The drugs' effects will compound the person's inability to function. A history of one or more surgical interventions for pain relief can be elicited, and the possibility of postsurgical discomfort must be considered.

Feelings of increasing hopelessness and discouragement along with demoralization and loss of self-esteem are evident in the CIBPS patient. The negative tone and the patient's unhappy situation lead to increasingly poor relationships with family and friends. Conflicts with and bitterness toward medical care personnel are fairly common because a cure is not achieved. Over time, the physical condition also worsens. A fear of hurting oneself, an unwillingness to be active, and an increased preoccupation with the sick role may end in a bedridden, withdrawn state.

CAUSATION

How can a person arrive at a state so distressing and disabling? Numerous pathways exist that transform a relatively well and adequately functioning individual into a helpless, long-suffering creature.

1. Our medical retirement and compensation systems sometimes are an incentive for perpetuating pain behavior. Following some relatively minor injury, a patient will proceed to manifest increasing pain and disability until he or she is rated "totally disabled." Once this state is achieved, it is made permanent because the patient believes he or she must continue to demonstrate invalid status, or because the system requires it with annual physical examinations. Certain physicians and lawyers may provide support for the patient's decision to go for total disability retirement. Naturally, a strong disincentive to get better exists during and after litigation.

2. The complaints of persistent pain in the absence of appropriate physical findings are often a result of the secondary gain the patient achieves from being disabled. A psychological conflict may be uncovered that is temporarily related to the onset of the pain. Alternatively, the pain solves a life problem that is distasteful, or it provides an acceptable way for dependency needs to be met.

3. At times the complications of CIBPS become part of a complex psychophysical pattern. The patient may be toxic from prescribed depressant drugs. He or she may have some drug-drug interaction because of simultaneous treatment by a number of doctors. A chronic arachnoiditis or other sequel to surgery for the pain may cause pain in its own right. In the desperate search for relief, a number of "healers" may have treated or maltreated the patient.

4. Although malingering or chronic factitious disorders can produce similar symptomatology, they are not considered here.

MANAGEMENT

Instead of an increasing preoccupation with pain, the major effort is to engage the patient in nonpain-oriented thinking. In addition, conditioning is reversed so that non-pain behavior is rewarded, and pain is set aside as a central focus of existence. A wide variety of modalities can be used to deal with chronic pain.

Patient education is helpful in explaining the nature of pain and the influence of mental attitudes in its control. Sometimes fears about the meaning of pain make the suffering more intense and these fears should be explored and clarified.

A deliberate program of increasing, rather than decreasing, activity is important. Physical therapy and exercise commensurate with the patient's ability and needs are instituted so that ways to function can be learned. If retraining for a more sedentary job is necessary, occupational therapy and vocational retraining will teach and practice ways to perform within one's capabilities. The patient must assume an active role in rehabilitation.

Relaxation techniques are worthwhile and helpful for reducing pain, inducing sleep, and achieving internal calm. Biofeedback, progressive relaxation exercises, and self-hypnosis are methods for achieving the relaxed state. Adequate support systems, especially families instructed to encourage the patient to function within his or her capabilities, are needed. The family should be taught that pain behavior is emitted from their cues and from others in the patient's environment. They cannot reward the sick or the pain role in CIBPS patients who are close to them.

Some general principles of pharmacotherapy include not using injectable medications for chronic pain and not prescribing "as needed" medication. PRN orders fix the patient's attention on the anticipation of pain. Ideally, regular oral medication will defuse the patient's concern about missing a dose. Naturally, a fixed schedule of analgesia will require reduced amounts of the medication. If the pain occurs only at certain times of the day, then medication should be offered only at these times. Employing the nonpharmacologic therapies mentioned, a fair number of patients will require no analgesic medication at all. Narcotics are often not needed. From what has been mentioned under "causation," it is evident that narcotics can do little to relieve the CIBPS. When narcotics are appropriate, the second-tier narcotics like codeine combined with a nonnarcotic analgesic are preferred. As many as half the patients arrive at the office or clinic already dependent on a narcotic or sedative. They should be detoxified and will often report that they feel better or, at least, mentally clearer than when overmedicated.

The triad of pain-depression-insomnia is a common one. Dealing with the insomnia and the depression will reduce complaints of pain. The sedative antihistamines, hydroxyzine, and the benzodiazepines are sometimes needed to supplement the nocturnal sedation. The tricyclic antidepressants, especially those with a sedative quality, can be given at bedtime for insomnia, depression, and secondary pain relief. Tegretol and Dilantin are drugs that give good antinociceptive results in certain cases, usually when a central pain component is present.

It is now known that certain cutaneous stimuli induce a degree of analgesia. Stimulation-produced analgesia works over the endorphin system or via the various spinal and medullary gates that can modulate pain. It also elevates pain thresholds, perhaps by altering neurotransmitter levels. So there are multiple mechanisms for environmental stimuli to successfully reduce pain, some of which can be reversed by the narcotic antagonist naloxone (Narcan). For example, acupuncture analgesia is blocked by naloxone, although this finding is still not fully confirmed. In animals, foot shock releases endogenous opioids and naloxone blocks the analgesia. Stimulation-produced analgesia is not simply a stress response. Some stimuli evoke it; other equally stressful stimuli do not.

An observation dating back to Hippocrates shows that counterirritation alleviates pain. It seems to be based on endogenous opioid production, gating, or both. An example of counterirritation is ice massages used in a number of pain clinics. Pain relief lasts for a time after the massage is completed. Transcutaneous electrical stimulation is another method of dermal stimulation that diminishes pain, acute and chronic. Implantable neural stimulators probably work over similar mechanisms of stimulation-produced analgesia.

Innumerable instances of "disattention" to pain can be cited. These may have a scientific basis in one of the above-mentioned mechanisms for modulating pain. Focusing on the pain, as many CIBPS patients do, will intensify it, and every effort must be made to divert their attention and train them to concentrate on other areas, like work or play.

DISCUSSION

It is difficult, sometimes impossible, to treat a CIBPS patient when disability litigation is under way. Ideally, such a person should have been helped to prevent the syndrome years earlier. Even though financial security and lack of the need to compete for a job are very considerable gains, the subsequent life of invalidism is too high a price to pay.

CIBPS patients should learn the difference between a handicap and a disability. A significant minority of our work force performs under substantial handicaps, including pain. CIBPS patients believe they are disabled. When they come to the conclusion that they are only handicapped, their existence becomes much more bearable and rewarding.

BIBLIOGRAPHY

- Brown, R.M., Pinkert, T.M. and Ludford, J.P. (Eds) Contemporary Research in Pain and Analgesia, 1983. NIDA Research Monograph 45.

Supt. of Documents, U.S. Government Printing Office, Washington, D.C. 20402.

- Ng, L.K.Y. (Ed) New approaches to the treatment of chronic pain: A review of multidisciplinary pain clinics and pain centers. NIDA Research Monograph 36, 1981. Supt. of Documents, U.S. Government Printing Office, Washington, D.C. 20402

53. Differential Diagnosis of Substance Abuse Symptoms and Signs

Often, the person with a drug disorder appears at the hospital with a condition for which there is no obvious diagnosis of the drug or drugs responsible. Instead, he or she presents with a number of subjective complaints or abnormalities. This information must be differentiated, not only from the specific drugs that may be involved, but also from medical conditions unrelated to drug disorders. In the following attempt to unravel the diagnostic tangles, a number of the nondrug induced conditions will be mentioned; many others would have to be considered as well.

INTOXICATION

A temporary distortion of cerebral functioning due to recent ingestion of a psychotropic drug usually resulting in maladaptive behavior. Two types can be identified, those with cerebellar signs (ataxia, slurred speech, nystagmus, incoordination) and those without cerebellar involvement.

Cerebellar Type Intoxification

1. alcohol
2. sedative-hypnotics
3. volatile solvents
4. anticholinergics
5. phencyclidine
6. opiates
7. bromides

Without Cerebellar Signs

1. stimulants
2. hallucinogens
3. cannabis

A large number of medical conditions can result in intoxication, including dehydration, oxygen insufficiency, electrolytic distortions, and reduced cerebral blood flow. In addition, digitalis, certain antibiotics, and steroids are some medicines that can intoxicate.

COMA

Drug Induced

1. opiate overdose
2. sedative-hypnotic overdose
3. alcohol overdose
4. phencyclidine overdose
5. volatile solvent overdose
6. anticholinergic overdose

Nondrug Induced

1. brain injury or disease
2. hypoglycemia
3. diabetic acidosis
4. hepatic coma
5. uremia
6. epilepsy

CONVULSIONS

Drug Induced

1. amphetamines
2. cocaine
3. lidocaine (cocaine adulterant)
4. phencyclidine
5. neuroleptics
6. LSD (rare)
7. meperidine in high doses

8. opiates (infrequent)
9. alcohol withdrawal
10. Ts and blues (Talwin and pyribenzamine)

Nondrug Induced

1. epilepsy, primary and secondary
2. uremia
3. fever in children
4. lead poisoning
5. anoxia
6. eclampsia

PSYCHOSIS (schizophreniform)

Drug Induced

1. amphetamines
2. cocaine
3. hallucinogens
4. phencyclidine
5. cannabis in high doses
6. alcohol hallucinosis
7. sedative-hypnotic withdrawal, atypical

Nondrug Induced

1. schizophrenia
2. affective disorders
3. organic mental disorders
4. paranoid disorders
5. borderline states
6. mental retardation
7. Cushing's syndrome

CEREBRAL HEMORRHAGE

Drug Induced

1. amphetamines (acute hypertension)
2. cocaine (acute hypertension)
3. phencyclidine (acute hypertension)

Nondrug Induced

1. congenital aneurysm
2. arteriosclerotic cerebrovascular disease
3. trauma

SUICIDE

Drug Induced

1. alcohol (during intoxication and withdrawal)
2. sedative-hypnotics (also means of suicide)
3. postcocaine depression
4. postamphetamine depression
5. reserpine
6. steroids
7. tricyclic antidepressants (means of suicide)

Nondrug Induced

1. affective disorders
2. organic depressive syndrome
3. schizophrenia
4. schizoaffective disorders
5. chronic painful physical illness
6. situational depression

HOMICIDE

Drug Induced

1. alcohol, including pathological intoxication
2. phencyclidine
3. sedative-hypnotic disorders
4. amphetamines
5. hallucinogens (rare)

Nondrug Induced

1. paranoid disorders
2. explosive disorders
3. antisocial personality disorders
4. paranoid schizophrenia

PUPILLARY DILATION (mydriasis)

Drug Induced

1. hallucinogens
2. amphetamines
3. cocaine
4. anticholinergics
5. opiate withdrawal
6. opiate overdose with anoxia
7. adrenalin

Nondrug Induced

1. anger
2. anxiety
3. glaucoma
4. occulomotor paralysis
5. subdural hematoma

CONSTRICTED PUPILS (miosis)

Drug Induced

1. opiates
2. pilocarpine
3. physostigmine

Nondrug Induced

1. brain stem lesions
2. CNS syphilis
3. syringomyelia

NYSTAGMUS (lateral eye flicks)

Drug Induced

1. alcohol intoxication
2. postalcohol state (nystagmus opposite in direction)
3. phencyclidine (may also be vertical)
4. sedative-hypnotics
5. phenytoin

Nondrug Induced

1. multiple sclerosis
2. syringomyelia
3. labyrinthitis

ANOREXIA (loss of appetite)

Drug Induced

1. amphetamines
2. amphetamine-like anoretics
3. cocaine
4. hallucinogens
5. alcohol intoxication
6. alcohol withdrawal
7. sedative-hypnotic withdrawal
8. opiate withdrawal
9. cannabis withdrawal

Nondrug Induced

1. malignancies
2. severe febrile illness
3. hepatitis
4. gastritis
5. depression
6. grief reactions
7. anorexia nervosa

TACHYCARDIA

Drug Induced

1. anticholinergics
2. cannabis
3. amphetamines
4. cocaine
5. hallucinogens
6. alcohol
7. phencyclidine
8. alcohol withdrawal

9. sedative-hypnotic withdrawal
10. opiate withdrawal

Nondrug Induced

1. thyrotoxicosis
2. febrile conditions
3. paroxysmal tachycardias
4. shock
5. hemorrhage
6. exertion
7. fever

CATATONIA (stupor, negativism, rigidity, posturing, stereotyped behavior or excitement)

Drug Induced

1. amphetamine ("overamping")
2. cocaine
3. phencyclidine
4. organic fluorides
5. hallucinogens (rare)

Nondrug Induced

1. catatonic schizophrenia
2. encephalitis
3. hepatic encephalopathy
4. dissociative disorders
5. mid-brain lesions

BRADYCARDIA

Drug Induced

1. opiates
2. digitalis

Nondrug Induced

1. heart block
2. jaundice
3. athletes' heart syndrome

CONFIRMATORY TESTS

The most direct and objective verification of one of the above diagnostic possibilities is clinical laboratory testing of the appropriate body fluid or breath. Cannabis (as THC metabolites), cocaine (as benzoylegconine), most opiates, many sedative-hypnotics, amphetamines, phencyclidine, and alcohol can be routinely tested for. Many laboratories are capable of studying tissues or body fluids for specific substances not routinely examined. Hundreds of toxic drugs and chemicals can be analyzed and detected in humans in larger laboratories.

MULTIPLE DRUGS AND MULTIPLE CAUSES

It is often difficult to make a precise clinical diagnosis of toxicity from a single drug. The problem becomes much more complicated when two or more drugs have been consumed. A person may be scratching for hallucinated parasites under the skin during a cocaine psychosis and also be stuporous from ingesting a large amount of methaqualone or diazepam.

Sometimes the obvious diagnosis may be incomplete or incorrect. A comatose man is brought into an emergency room. He reeks of alcohol and his BAL is .27 percent. He is treated for alcohol intoxication but his condition worsens. At autopsy a massive subdural hematoma is found, presumably the result of a fall during the intoxication. A woman is found in a coma from which she can be minimally aroused by painful stimulation. Alcohol is noted on her breath. It turns out that the coma is not due to alcohol but to diabetic ketoacidosis.

SYNERGISM

The list of diagnostic possibilities noted above can be used to determine whether two drugs will enhance each other's effect. For example, the use of cocaine and marijuana will accelerate the heart rate more than either drug alone. Another example: It has been shown that the ability of people to exercise maximally is diminished by prior smoking of marijuana because the drug can increase the heart rate 20 to 50 percent in the resting state. Exertion will add to the tachycardia. At a heart rate of about 160 beats per minute, cardiac efficiency begins to decrease.

SUMMARY

The signs and symptoms mentioned here form a partial list of the common physical and mental changes induced by certain drugs. The list may be helpful when considering the possibility that a certain drug is responsible for the clinical picture presented. Drug involvement is an important consideration in clarifying the cause of some obscure conditions in adolescents and young adults.

54. A Matter of
Quality Control:
Manufactured Drugs of Abuse

The adulteration of illicit drugs is a familiar story. Nobody expects heroin to be pure heroin or cocaine to be pure cocaine. In fact, if 100 percent heroin or cocaine were suddenly to become available, it would be disastrous since the material at the retail level has a fraction of the potency. Poisonings and overdoses would flood urban emergency services.

Contamination is another fact of life-and-death on the street. More than 85 percent of needle users test positive for hepatitis B. Localized and blood stream infections are fairly common complications. Some of the bacteria, viruses, and fungi are introduced into the product during its cursory preparation for sale. Users' unsterile techniques introduce additional spores, protozoans, and other microorganisms into their veins.

When underground entrepreneurs take it upon themselves to produce synthetic illegal drugs accidentally or deliberately, serious toxic reactions can be sold to an unprotected, even uncaring, consumer market. During Prohibition (1920-1933) the use of lead-containing equipment by bootleggers caused cases of encephalitis and polyneuritis in some imbibers. If ethanol was in short supply, methanol (wood alcohol) was substituted without qualms. In sufficient amounts methanol causes irreversible blindness.

More recently, a few rash chemists have come forth with concoctions that turned out to be not quite what were intended. Instead of PCP, some batches have been found to contain the carbonitrile of phencyclidine (PCC). This analogue causes violent gastrointestinal reactions fore and aft with a few fatal terminations.

Although inexperience or poor equipment may induce such inept chemical misadventures, some of it is due to a lack of concern for the consumer. The buyer is a few levels removed from the would-be or actual chemist, and little motivation exists to turn out a safe and genuine product. One tragic chemical error has recently emphasized the hazardous nature of using other-than-legal drugs.

310

MPPP
(1-methyl-4-phenyl-proprionoxy-piperidine)

MPPP is a synthetic narcotic structurally related to meperidine (Demerol). Meperidine is 1-methyl-4-phenylnipecotate. MPPP is used in the manufacture of certain industrial chemicals. It is not controlled at present.

In 1977 a 23-year-old graduate student in chemistry attempted to synthesize MPPP in his laboratory, apparently for personal use. He decided to simplify the synthesis, but in so doing, converted some of the material to MPTP. Shortly after using some of the contaminated material, he developed symptoms of severe Parkinsonism and was so diagnosed by Dr. Davis at the University of Tennessee. The next year the chemist managed to overdose with some unknown drug and died. This event provided an opportunity for an autopsy. It was found that he had, indeed, been suffering from Parkinsonism because the cellular components of the substantia nigra in the extrapyramidal system of the brain were few and far between. The case report was published in *Psychiatry Research* in 1978 after Dr. Davis had moved to the National Institute of Mental Health.

MPTP
(1-methyl-4-phenyl-1, 2, 5, 6-tetrahydropyridine)

MPTP is a neurotoxin that damages and kills neurons in the substantia nigra and probably affects other neuronal systems.

The pars compacta of the substantia is a dopamine factory for the corpus striatum. It conveys dopamine along neuronal axons to the striatal area of the brain where posture and muscle tone are controlled. A lack of dopamine in this extrapyramidal structure will cause rigidity and other signs of the extrapyramidal syndrome (EPS). Individuals with Parkinsonism ordinarily show degenerative changes in the substantia nigra and related structures. Patients who take dopamine blockers like neuroleptics frequently manifest a Parkinson-like syndrome early in treatment. After months or years of antipsychotic therapy a tardive dyskinesia can emerge.

The story of the erstwhile chemist who synthesized the wrong compound would hardly be worth telling were it not for a similar blunder in northern California which had more widespread consequences. In the San Francisco Bay area about 200 people have advanced Parkinson's disease or have the possibility of developing it as they age.

It is remarkable that a single injection of MPTP can produce a picture identical with Parkinsonism. Some of the common manifestations of the EPS are rigidity, a pill-rolling tremor, a fixed, blank facial expression, seborrhea, and eventually mental blunting. All movements are performed slowly and the posture is stooped. Its cause is unknown. Since Parkinsonism occurs in the elderly, the diagnosis of the condition in young adults is difficult. The last time young people had the condition in large numbers was during the postinfluenza encephalitis epidemic of 1918–1920. Carbon monoxide poisoning can also leave a patient with the EPS. Both conditions affect the substantia nigra.

MPTP produces Parkinsonism so specifically that some clinicians are wondering whether this drug or some related substance is the cause of the disease. A few chemists who have used the drug during industrial operations have come down with the same movement disorders, presumably from inhaling it or by absorption through the skin.

It was during the summer of 1982 that a narcotic addict appeared at the Santa Clara Medical Center in San Jose unable to move or talk. Since he was only 42 years old, a diagnosis of Parkinsonism was not seriously considered. However, a week later the addict's sister arrived at the clinic with a hand tremor, a blank stare, and slow movements of the extremities and trunk. At this time the neurologists Langston and Ballard elicited the history that the siblings had purchased a new "synthetic heroin" from their dealer. It was shortly after using the material that the characteristic symptoms appeared. A small amount of the drug was still available, and it was sent to a few laboratories for analysis and identification.

According to an article by Robert Lewin in the June 8, 1984 issue of *Science*, Dr. Ballard happened to meet Dr. Tetrud, a neurologist from Watsonville, about 50 miles south of San Jose. Dr. Tetrud mentioned the strange case of two young brothers with muscle rigidity that produced immobility. It turned out that these two were also opiate dependent and had recently used some "synthetic heroin." It was from information of this sort and from the steady flow of similar patients into the Santa Clara Valley clinic that a diagnosis of chemically induced Parkinsonism could be made.

But what was the chemical? The laboratories had difficulties identifying the structural formula. Fortunately, the toxicologist at one of the laboratories remembered the 1979 *Psychiatric Research* article by Davis et al. about MPTP. Immediately, the analytic chemists could determine that the northern California miniepidemic was caused by the same chemical. Langston, Tetrud, and Irwin, who finally identified the sample as MPTP, published their report in the February 23, 1983, issue of *Science*. Later the NIMH group published a paper indicating that MPTP produces a model of Parkinsonism in monkeys.

The San Jose physicians alerted the public through media announcements about the dangerous "synthetic heroin" sold on the street. It is estimated that 200–300 heroin users have exposed themselves to the drug and a few additional people come forth each month. Dr. Langston speculates that those who remain asymptomatic at present may be vulnerable to Parkinsonism in their late years since the aging process seems to provide an additional burden upon the dopamine system.

DISCUSSION

The MPTP story abounds in paradoxes, coincidences, and opportunities, to say nothing of tragedies.

- To look up the synthesis of MPTP, Dr. Langston went to the Stanford library where he discovered the 1947 paper by Ziering, and subsequent articles about making MPTP were cut out of the bound volumes. It seems likely the supplier of the material had used the library as reference and didn't want to leave it around for future avaricious chemists.

- During the 1950s a pharmaceutical firm actually did a small pilot study of MPTP as a potential *anti*-Parkinson drug because of its resemblance to certain neurotransmitters. Of course, it didn't work.

- Does MPTP cause the sort of Parkinson's disease that comes with aging? It is so specific in its action that it is tempting to wonder whether this drug or something like it may enter the body in trace amounts over a lifetime. MPTP produces all signs of the disease including the seborrhea. Nevertheless, it is somewhat farfetched to assume that this product, which does not exist in nature, is causative. Other substantia nigra-specific chemicals may have an etiologic role in what was called "paralysis agitans" in the old textbooks. But the chemical would have to have a worldwide distribution.

- The culprit is not MPTP but a metabolite of it. If the oxidation of MPTP is blocked in primates, the disease will not be manifested. Interestingly, in Germany, amine oxidase inhibitors are part of the treatment of Parkinsonism.

- What of the patients? Some of them have acute, fulminating Parkinsonism, a serious condition hardly seen before. They require large amounts of dopamine agonists and of L-DOPA to keep alive. A few people might see this tragedy as an argument to legalize the distribution of opiates so that incidents such as the MPTP syndrome can be avoided. It may be claimed that drug-dependent individuals have the right to quality, purified material to support their addiction. Realistically, it is impossible to protect persons who will not take the responsibility for protecting themselves. In England where heroin addicts are given sterile opiates and syringes, the incidence of hepatitis and bloodstream infections matches ours. Sterile use still requires sterile water, sterile preparation, and sterile injection techniques. Addicts tend to be careless or uncaring about these matters. Instead, the MPTP episode tells us that we must be careful of what we introduce into our bodies. The makers and providers of illicit drugs have no interest in sanitation, accuracy, or quality control, and they are not to be trusted.

Internal pollution is worse than environmental pollution. In the first instance the poison is introduced in concentrated form and by oneself. Those who inject, smoke, or swallow dubious substances have no self-esteem, no concept of future consequences, and are extremely immature or self-destructive.

- What of the chemist who developed this "synthetic heroin"? He must be aware of the havoc he caused. Hopefully, he has ceased perpetuating the disaster. If he has, others will still discover the same flawed process. It is hoped that victims of this ignoble chemical "experiment" have identified the dealer or dealers. This should easily lead back to the source of these misbegotten molecules.

- The symptoms of MPTP Parkinsonism are so severe that large doses of bromocriptine and L-DOPA are needed to reduce the rigidity that can interfere with eating, drinking, and speech.

- The only visible benefit from the gloomy MPTP tale is that an animal model for Parkinson's disease is now available. This will reawaken interest in this condition and we can expect new knowledge and improved treatments in the future.

- Parkinsonism should not be confused with acute catatonic schizophrenia.

Index

WITHDRAWN